God's greatest desire is for us to live victorious lives and continually enjoy his blessings bequeathed to us. As God is Spirit & Man also is a Spirit so Walk in divine excellence and transform your world through the power of a renewed mind.

Contents

Symbol	Disease, Symptoms, Risk factor & Natural Remedy
A	Male Infertility
B	Oligospermia
C	Male Hypogonadism
D	Gynecomastia
E	Testicular Disease
F	Testicular Cancer
G	Prostate Cancer
H	BPH
I	Varicocele
J	Hydrocele
K	Inflammation of the Testicle (Orchitis)
L	Epididymitis
M	Spermatorrhoea

Male Infertility

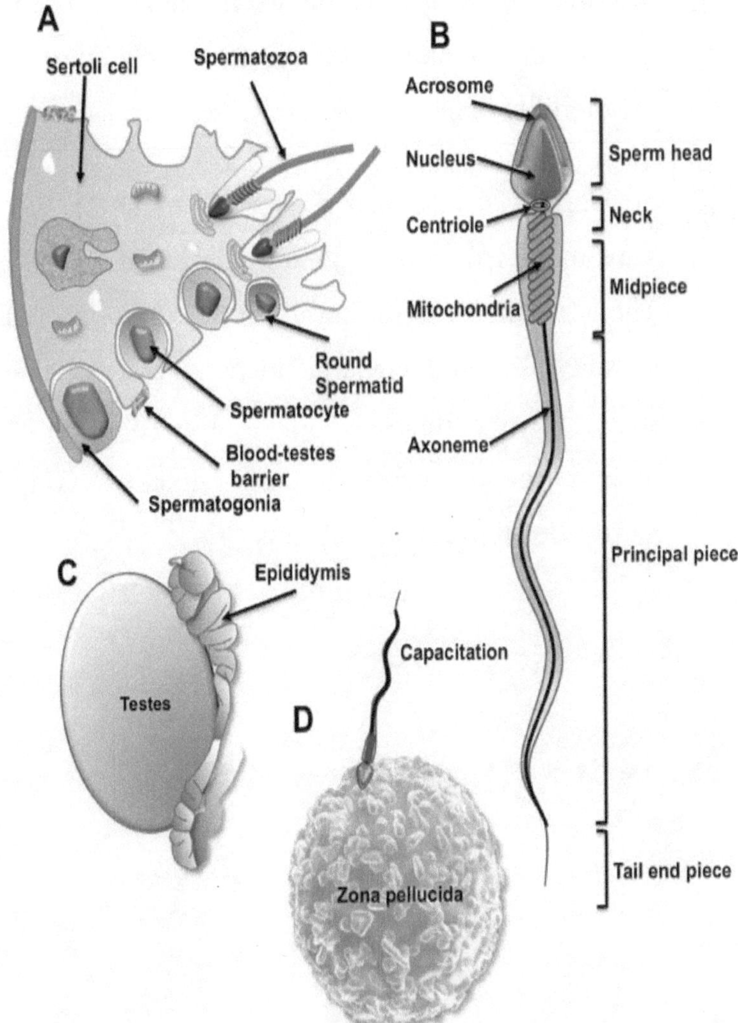

Although some people still think of fertility as a "woman's problem," in 20% of infertile couples, the problem is solely with the male partner. Infertility in a man may be the only reason that a couple can't conceive, or it may simply add to the difficulties caused by infertility in his partner.

So it's crucial that men get tested for fertility as well as women. It's also important that men do it early. Though some guys may want to put off being tested -- possibly to avoid embarrassment -- early testing can spare their partners a great deal of unnecessary discomfort and expense. It's also a good way to quickly narrow down potential problems.

Getting Tested for Infertility

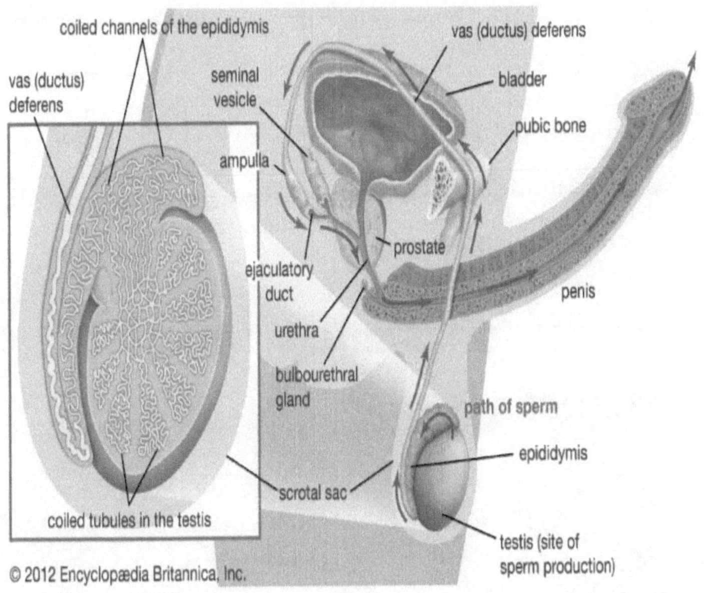

The first thing to do for fertility issues is to go to the doctor, typically a urologist. After a physical exam, your doctor will probably order a semen analysis, which will check the quality and quantity of the sperm in the semen. And yes, your doctor will want you to give the sample there, or at least someplace nearby, because it's important that the analysis takes place quickly. Just remember, as sheepish as you might feel, a semen analysis is a common test, and the results could save you months of worry and stress.

If the first semen analysis is normal, your doctor may order a second test to confirm the results. Two normal tests usually are interpreted to mean that the man doesn't have any significant infertility problems. If something in the results looks irregular, your doctor might order further tests to pinpoint the problem. At this point, if you aren't already seeing a urologist, you should considering seeing a specialist.

What a Semen Analysis Can Detect

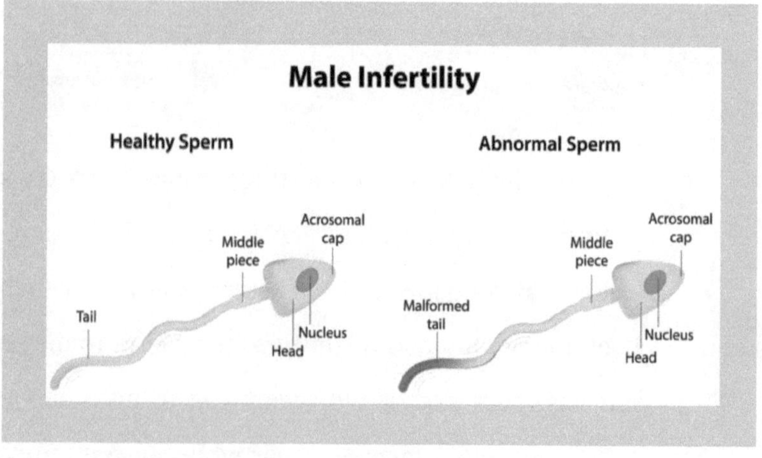

- Azoospermia. No sperm are produced, or the sperm aren't appearing in the semen.
- Oligospermia. Few sperm are produced.

- Problems with sperm motility; if sperm aren't moving normally, they are less likely to be capable of fertilizing an egg.
- Problems with sperm morphology; problems with the form and structure -- or morphology -- of the sperm may cause infertility.

But while these conditions may be the direct reason that you can't conceive, they themselves may be caused by an underlying medical condition. Your doctor will probably want to investigate the issue further by ordering blood and urine tests or other procedures.

Reasons for Male Infertility

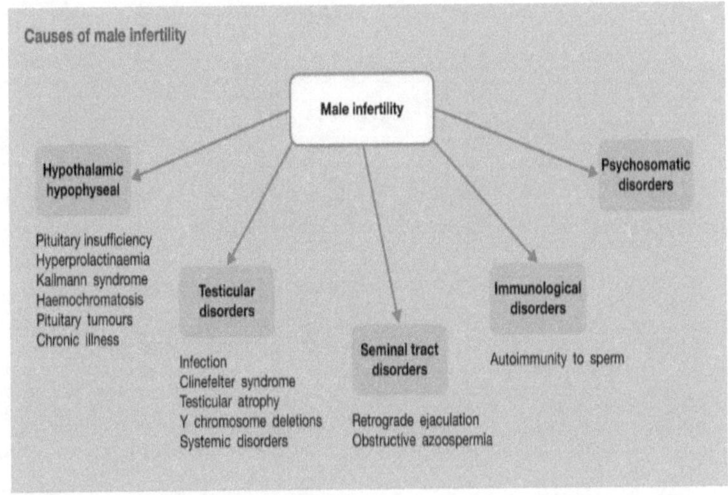

There are a wide number of reasons for male infertility. Some are caused by physical problems that prevent the sperm from being ejaculated normally in semen. Others affect the quality and production of the sperm itself.

Possible Male Fertility Problem

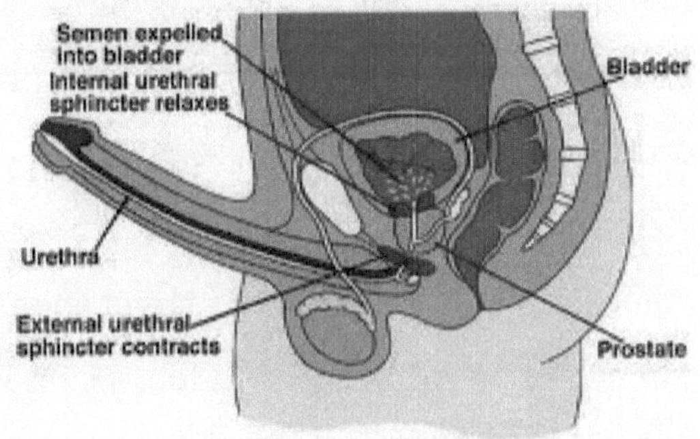

- Sexually transmitted diseases or other infections. Genital infections such as chlamydia and gonorrhea can cause infertility in men. The infertility can often be resolved by treating the infection.

- Blockages, birth defects, or physical damage. In some cases, men are born with blockages in parts of the testicle or other abnormalities that prevent sperm from getting into the semen. Physical trauma to the testicles, prostate, and urethra can also result in fertility problems. Surgery can sometimes correct the problem.

- Retrograde ejaculation. In this disorder, semen doesn't come out of the penis during ejaculation, but instead enters the bladder. It can be caused by diabetes, certain medications, and surgery to the bladder, prostate, or urethra.

- Genetic diseases. Although it's rare, genetic illnesses such as cystic fibrosis or chromosomal disorders can cause infertility.

- Autoimmune problems. In some cases, the immune system can mistakenly target sperm cells and treat them as if they were a foreign virus. The sperm can become damaged as a result.

- Hormonal problems. Certain hormonal imbalances -- in the pituitary and thyroid glands, for instance -- can cause infertility. Your doctor may suggest treatment with medication.

- Sexual problems. Erectile dysfunction (impotence) and premature ejaculation can obviously have an effect on fertility. Erectile dysfunction can be caused by psychological problems such as anxiety, guilt, or low self-esteem. It is also caused by physical problems such as diabetes, high blood pressure, high cholesterol, and heart disease. In addition, impotence may be a side effect of certain medications such as antidepressants. Talk to your doctor about ways of treating any sexual problems.

- Varicoceles. Varicoceles are enlarged varicose veins that develop in the scrotum and prevent blood from flowing properly. Varicoceles are found in 15% of all men and in up to 40% of men being evaluated for infertility. Although they may be a factor in male infertility, recent studies question whether surgery to correct varicoceles has any beneficial effect.

Other Factors in Male Infertility

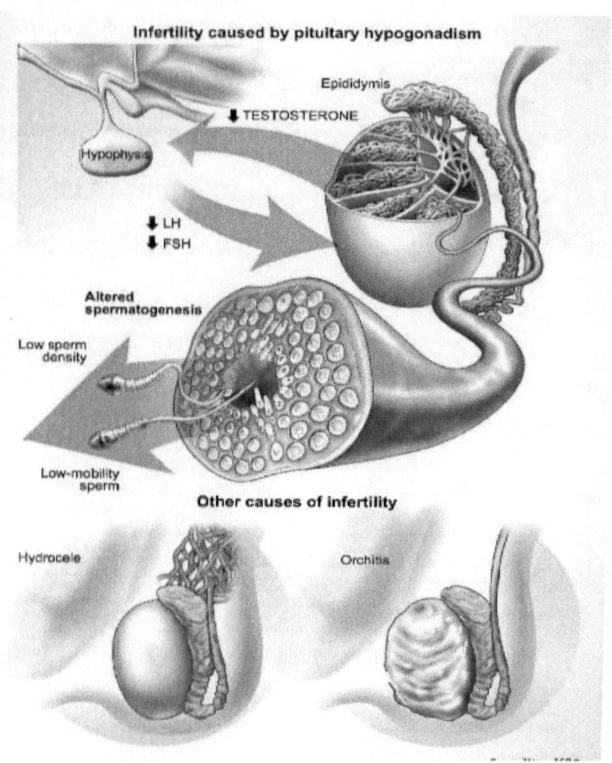

- Excessive exercise; studies have shown that exercising too much may lead to the release of too many steroid hormones. This can affect fertility.
- Stress
- Obesity

- Use of drugs such as marijuana and cocaine, taking steroids, drinking alcohol, and smoking can reduce sperm counts.

- Exposure to toxins and environmental hazards; pesticides, lead, radiation, radioactive substances, mercury, and heavy metals may affect fertility.

- Heat; although the effect is usually temporary, high temperatures in the testicles could reduce sperm production. High heat could result from wearing clothing that's too tight and traps heat, frequent bike riding, or by taking too many hot baths or saunas.

Getting Pregnant With Male Infertility

If you're a guy who has been diagnosed with infertility, you should talk to your doctor about any behavioral changes you can make that might increase your chances of conceiving.

If your sperm count is low, your doctor may recommend having intercourse less frequently in order to build up a better concentration of sperm. You should also ask about taking vitamins. Some recent studies have found that men can improve their low sperm counts by taking a combination of a folic acid and zinc.

If you have abnormal hormone levels, your doctor may recommend hormone treatment.

If you have retrograde ejaculation, you can often treat this with common over-the-counter cold medicine.

In some cases where the man has mild infertility, artificial insemination or other assisted reproduction techniques, such as GIFT, ZIFT or IVF, may be helpful. One exciting treatment for male infertility and low sperm count is a form of micromanipulation called intracytoplasmic sperm injection (ICSI). This is a laboratory procedure in which sperm and eggs are retrieved from both partners, and then a single sperm is injected into an egg. The fertilized egg is then implanted into the woman's uterus.

If the man doesn't have sperm in his semen, one of several techniques can be used to retrieve sperm from the testicles. Success rates are generally good -- as high as 65% in some clinics. But factors such as poor sperm quality, poor egg quality, and the older age of the mother can lessen the chance of success. Other techniques that might help men with fertility problems are being developed.

What is Oligospermia?

Oligospermia is a male fertility issue characterized by a low sperm count. Other aspects of the sexual health of men with this condition are typical. This includes the ability to get and maintain an erection, as well as produce ejaculation at orgasm.

Sperm count in your ejaculate can vary throughout your life. A healthy sperm amount is often necessary for fertility. The World Health Organization (WHO) classifies sperm counts at or above 15 million sperm per milliliter (mL) of semen as average. Anything below that is considered low and is diagnosed as oligospermia.

- Mild oligospermia is 10 to 15 million sperm/mL.

- Moderate oligospermia is considered 5 to 10 million sperm/mL.

- Severe oligospermia is diagnosed when sperm counts fall between 0 and 5 million sperm/mL.

It's unclear how many men have low sperm amounts in their semen. This is, in part, because not everyone with the condition is diagnosed. Only men who have difficulty with conceiving naturally and ultimately seek help may be diagnosed.

Causes

Several conditions and lifestyle factors can increase a man's risk for oligospermia.

Varicocele

Enlarged veins in a man's scrotum can disrupt blood flow to the testicles. This can cause the temperature in the testicles to increase. Any increase in temperature can negatively impact sperm production. About 40 percent of men with low sperm numbers or low sperm quality count have this common issue. Read more about varicocele.

Infection

Viruses like sexually transmitted infections can reduce the sperm amount in semen.

Ejaculation issues

While many men with oligospermia have typical ejaculations, some ejaculation problems may reduce sperm count. Retrograde ejaculation is one such issue. This occurs when semen enters the bladder instead of leaving from the tip of the penis.

Other things that may interfere with typical ejaculation include:

- injuries

- tumors

- cancer

- past surgeries

Hormone issues

The brain and the testicles produce several hormones that are responsible for ejaculation and sperm production. An imbalance in any of these hormones may lower sperm count numbers.

Exposure to chemicals and metals

Pesticides, cleaning agents, and painting materials are a few of the chemicals that can reduce sperm count. Exposure to heavy metals, such as lead, can cause this problem, too.

Overheating testicles

Sitting frequently, placing laptops over your genitals, and wearing tight clothing may all contribute to overheating. An increase in temperature around the testicles may temporarily reduce sperm production. It's unclear what long-term complications may occur.

Drug and alcohol use

The use of some substances, including marijuana and cocaine, may reduce sperm counts. Excessive drinking can do the same. Men who smoke cigarettes may have lower sperm counts than men who do not smoke.

Weight problems

Being overweight or obese increases your risk for low sperm counts in several ways. Excess weight can directly reduce how much sperm your body can make. Weight problems may also interfere with hormone production.

How does oligospermia affect fertility?

Some men with oligospermia can still conceive despite lower sperm counts. Fertilization may be more difficult, however. It may take more attempts than couples without a fertility issue.

Other men with oligospermia may have no problem with conception, despite the low sperm numbers.

Some of the most common causes of oligospermia also increase a man's risk for other fertility issues. This includes sperm motility problems.

Sperm motility refers to how "active" sperm are in a man's semen. Normal activity allows sperm to swim toward an egg for fertilization easily. Abnormal motility may mean the sperm don't move enough to reach an egg. The sperm may also move in an unpredictable pattern that would prevent them from reaching an egg.

Most effective Homeopathic Treatment of Oligospermia

A. Type Composition :-

(Mix all the following Compositions of 20 ml in 100 ml File)

1.Ashwagandha Q

2. Damiana Q

3. Ginseng Q

4. Buforana Q (LM)

Dose:- 30 Drops with ½ Cup of Water 4 Times a Day

B. Take the followings with above Type A Composition

1. Lycopodium 200 CH (2 Drops Morning)

2. Thuja 200 CH (2 Drops Night)

3. Rhododendron 200 CH (2 Drops Noon)

Male Hypogonadism

Male hypogonadism is a condition in which the body doesn't produce enough testosterone — the hormone that plays a key role in masculine growth and development during puberty — or has an impaired ability to produce sperm or both.

You may be born with male hypogonadism, or it can develop later in life, often from injury or infection. The effects — and what you can do about them — depend on the cause and at what point in your life male hypogonadism occurs. Some types of male hypogonadism can be treated with testosterone replacement therapy.

Symptoms

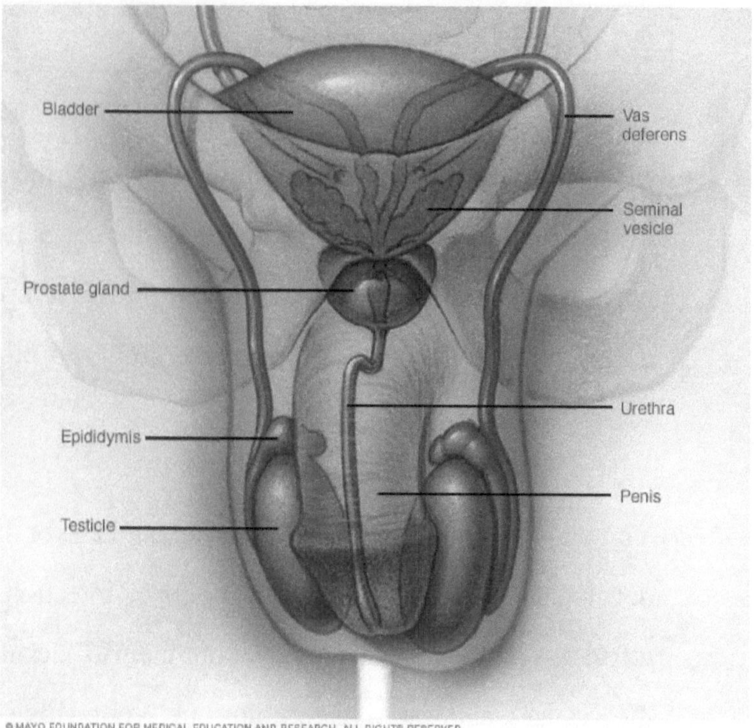

Male reproductive system

Hypogonadism can begin during fetal development, before puberty or during adulthood. Signs and symptoms depend on when the condition develops.

Fetal development

If the body doesn't produce enough testosterone during fetal development, the result may be impaired growth of the external sex organs. Depending on when hypogonadism develops and how much testosterone is present, a child who is genetically male may be born with:

- Female genitals

- Ambiguous genitals — genitals that are neither clearly male nor clearly female

- Underdeveloped male genitals

Puberty

Male hypogonadism may delay puberty or cause incomplete or lack of normal development. It can cause:

- Decreased development of muscle mass

- Lack of deepening of the voice

- Impaired growth of body hair

- Impaired growth of the penis and testicles

- Excessive growth of the arms and legs in relation to the trunk of the body

- Development of breast tissue (gynecomastia)

Adulthood

In adult males, hypogonadism may alter certain masculine physical characteristics and impair normal reproductive function. Signs and symptoms may include:

- Erectile dysfunction

- Infertility

- Decrease in beard and body hair growth

- Decrease in muscle mass

- Development of breast tissue (gynecomastia)

- Loss of bone mass (osteoporosis)

Hypogonadism can also cause mental and emotional changes. As testosterone decreases, some men may experience symptoms similar to those of menopause in women. These may include:

- Fatigue

- Decreased sex drive

- Difficulty concentrating

- Hot flashes

When to see a doctor

See a doctor if you have any symptoms of male hypogonadism. Establishing the cause of hypogonadism is an important first step to getting appropriate treatment.

Causes

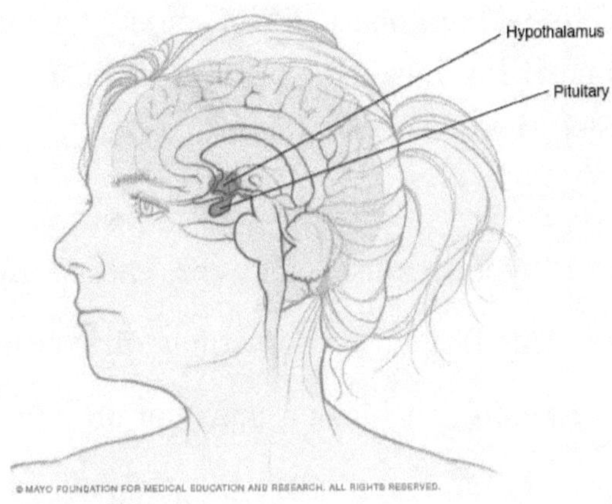

Pituitary gland and hypothalamus

Male hypogonadism means the testicles don't produce enough of the male sex hormone testosterone. There are two basic types of hypogonadism:

- **Primary.** This type of hypogonadism — also known as primary testicular failure — originates from a problem in the testicles.

- **Secondary.** This type of hypogonadism indicates a problem in the hypothalamus or the pituitary gland — parts of the brain that signal the testicles to produce testosterone. The hypothalamus produces gonadotropin-releasing hormone, which signals the pituitary gland to make follicle-stimulating hormone (FSH) and luteinizing hormone (LH). Luteinizing hormone then signals the testes to produce testosterone.

Either type of hypogonadism may be caused by an inherited (congenital) trait or something that happens later in life (acquired), such as an injury or an infection. At times, primary and secondary hypogonadism can occur together.

Primary hypogonadism

- Common causes of primary hypogonadism include:

- Klinefelter syndrome. This condition results from a congenital abnormality of the sex chromosomes, X and Y. A male normally has one X and one Y chromosome. In Klinefelter syndrome, two or more X chromosomes are present in addition to one Y chromosome. The Y chromosome contains the genetic material that determines the sex of a child and related development. The extra X chromosome that occurs in Klinefelter syndrome causes abnormal development of the testicles, which in turn results in underproduction of testosterone.

- Undescended testicles. Before birth, the testicles develop inside the abdomen and normally move down into their permanent place in the scrotum. Sometimes one or both of the testicles may not be descended at birth. This condition often corrects itself within the first few years of life without treatment. If not corrected in early childhood, it may lead to malfunction of the testicles and reduced production of testosterone.

- Mumps orchitis. If a mumps infection involving the testicles in addition to the salivary glands (mumps orchitis) occurs during adolescence or adulthood, long-term testicular damage may occur. This may affect normal testicular function and testosterone production.

- Hemochromatosis. Too much iron in the blood can cause testicular failure or pituitary gland dysfunction, affecting testosterone production.

- Injury to the testicles. Because they're situated outside the abdomen, the testicles are prone to injury. Damage to normally developed testicles can cause hypogonadism. Damage to one testicle may not impair total testosterone production.

- Cancer treatment. Chemotherapy or radiation therapy for the treatment of cancer can interfere with testosterone and sperm production. The effects of both treatments often are temporary, but permanent infertility may occur. Although many men regain their fertility within a few months after treatment ends, preserving sperm before starting cancer therapy is an option that many men consider.

Secondary hypogonadism

In secondary hypogonadism, the testicles are normal but function improperly due to a problem with the pituitary or hypothalamus. A number of conditions can cause secondary hypogonadism, including:

- Kallmann syndrome. Abnormal development of the hypothalamus — the area of the brain that controls the secretion of pituitary hormones — can cause hypogonadism. This abnormality is also associated with impaired development of the ability to smell (anosmia) and red-green color blindness.

- Pituitary disorders. An abnormality in the pituitary gland can impair the release of hormones from the pituitary gland to the testicles, affecting normal testosterone production. A pituitary tumor or other type of brain tumor located near the pituitary gland may cause testosterone or other hormone deficiencies. Also, the treatment for a brain tumor, such as surgery or radiation therapy, may impair pituitary function and cause hypogonadism.

- Inflammatory disease. Certain inflammatory diseases, such as sarcoidosis, histiocytosis and tuberculosis, involve the hypothalamus and pituitary gland and can affect testosterone production, causing hypogonadism.

- HIV/AIDS. HIV/AIDS can cause low levels of testosterone by affecting the hypothalamus, the pituitary and the testes.

- Medications. The use of certain drugs, such as opiate pain medications and some hormones, can affect testosterone production.

- Obesity. Being significantly overweight at any age may be linked to hypogonadism.

- Normal aging. Older men generally have lower testosterone levels than younger men do. As men age, there's a slow and continuous decrease in testosterone production.

- Concurrent illness. The reproductive system can temporarily shut down due to the physical stress of an illness or surgery, as well as during significant emotional stress. This is a result of diminished signals from the hypothalamus and usually resolves with successful treatment of the underlying condition.

The rate at which testosterone declines varies greatly among men. As many as 30 percent of men older than 75 have a testosterone level that's below the normal range of testosterone in young men. Whether treatment is necessary remains a matter of debate.

Risk factors

- Risk factors for hypogonadism include:

- Kallmann syndrome

- Undescended testicles as an infant

- Mumps infection affecting your testicles

- Injury to your testicles

- Testicular or pituitary tumors

- HIV/AIDS

- Klinefelter syndrome

- Hemochromatosis

- Previous chemotherapy or radiation therapy

- Untreated sleep apnea

Hypogonadism can be inherited. If any of these risk factors are in your family health history, tell your doctor.

- Complications

- The complications of untreated hypogonadism differ depending on what age it first develops — during fetal development, puberty or adulthood.

- Fetal development

- A baby may be born with:

- Ambiguous genitalia

- Abnormal genitalia

- Puberty

- Pubertal development can be delayed or incomplete, resulting in:

- Diminished or lack of beard and body hair

- Impaired penis and testicle growth

- Unproportional growth, usually increased length of arms and legs compared with the trunk

- Enlarged male breasts (gynecomastia)

- Adulthood

- Complications may include:

- Infertility

- Erectile dysfunction

- Decreased sex drive

- Fatigue

- Muscle loss or weakness

- Enlarged male breasts (gynecomastia)

- Decreased beard and body hair growth

- Osteoporosis

Most effective Homeopathic Treatment of Male Hypogonadism

1. Ashwagandha Q (20 Drops with ½ Cup of Water 4 Times A Day)

2. Testis Siccati 3X (Reckeweg) – 2 Pills 3 Times

3. Caladium Seguinum 30 CH – 2 Drops Morning

Gynecomastia

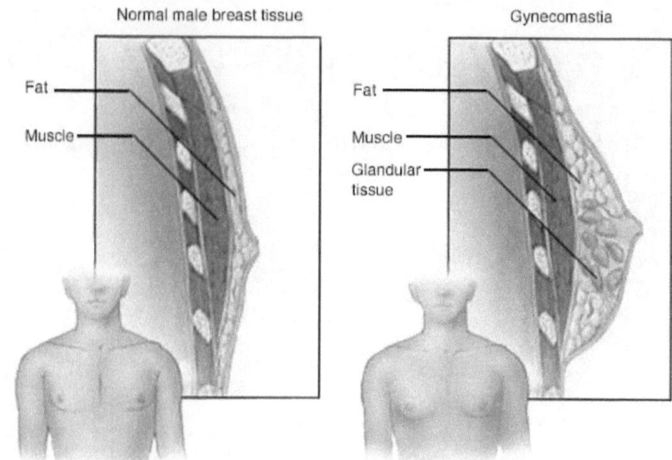

Enlarged breasts in men (gynecomastia)

Gynecomastia (guy-nuh-koh-MAS-tee-uh) is an increase in the amount of breast gland tissue in boys or men, caused by an imbalance of the hormones estrogen and testosterone. Gynecomastia can affect one or both breasts, sometimes unevenly.

Newborns, boys going through puberty and older men may develop gynecomastia as a result of normal changes in hormone levels, though other causes also exist.

Generally, gynecomastia isn't a serious problem, but it can be tough to cope with the condition. Men and boys with gynecomastia sometimes have pain in their breasts and may feel embarrassed.

Gynecomastia may go away on its own. If it persists, medication or surgery may help.

Symptoms

Signs and symptoms of gynecomastia include:

- Swollen breast tissue

- Breast tenderness

When to see a doctor

See your doctor if you have:

- Swelling

- Pain or tenderness

- Nipple discharge in one or both breasts

Causes

Gynecomastia is triggered by a decrease in the amount of the hormone testosterone compared with estrogen. The decrease can be caused by conditions that block the effects of testosterone, reduce testosterone or increase your estrogen level.

Several things can upset the hormone balance, including the following.

Natural hormone changes

The hormones testosterone and estrogen control sex characteristics in both men and women. Testosterone controls male traits, such as muscle mass and body hair. Estrogen controls female traits, including the growth of breasts.

Most people think of estrogen as an exclusively female hormone, but men also produce it — though normally in small quantities. Male estrogen levels that are too high or are out of balance with testosterone levels can cause gynecomastia.

- **Gynecomastia in infants.** More than half of male infants are born with enlarged breasts due to the effects of their mother's estrogen. Generally, the swollen breast tissue goes away within two to three weeks after birth.

- **Gynecomastia during puberty.** Gynecomastia caused by hormone changes during puberty is relatively common. In most cases, the swollen breast tissue will go away without treatment within six months to two years.

- **Gynecomastia in adults.** The prevalence of gynecomastia peaks again between the ages of 50 and 69. At least 1 in 4 men in this age group is affected.

Substances that can cause gynecomastia include:

- Alcohol

- Amphetamines, used to treat attention-deficit/hyperactivity disorder

- Marijuana

- Heroin

- Methadone (Methadose, Dolophine)

Health conditions

Several health conditions can cause gynecomastia by affecting the normal balance of hormones. These include:

- **Hypogonadism.** Conditions that interfere with normal testosterone production, such as Klinefelter syndrome or pituitary insufficiency, can be associated with gynecomastia.

- **Aging.** Hormone changes that occur with normal aging can cause gynecomastia, especially in men who are overweight.

- **Tumors.** Some tumors, such as those involving the testes, adrenal glands or pituitary gland, can produce hormones that alter the male-female hormone balance.

- **Hyperthyroidism.** In this condition, the thyroid gland produces too much of the hormone thyroxine.

- **Kidney failure.** About half the people being treated with dialysis experience gynecomastia due to hormonal changes.

- **Liver failure and cirrhosis.** Changes in hormone levels related to liver problems and cirrhosis medications are associated with gynecomastia.

- **Malnutrition and starvation.** When your body is deprived of adequate nutrition, testosterone levels drop while estrogen levels remain the same, causing a hormonal imbalance. Gynecomastia can also happen when normal nutrition resumes.

Herbal products

Plant oils, such as tea tree or lavender, used in shampoos, soaps or lotions have been associated with gynecomastia. This is probably due to their weak estrogenic activity.

Risk factors

Risk factors for gynecomastia include:

- Adolescence

- Older age

- Use of anabolic steroids or androgens to enhance athletic performance

- Certain health conditions, including liver and kidney disease, thyroid disease, hormonally active tumors, and Klinefelter syndrome

Complications

Gynecomastia has few physical complications, but it can cause psychological or emotional problems caused by appearance.

Prevention

There are a few factors you can control that may reduce the risk of gynecomastia:

- **Don't use drugs.** Examples include steroids and androgens, amphetamines, heroin, and marijuana.

- **Avoid alcohol.** Don't drink alcohol. If you do drink, do so in moderation.

- **Review your medications.** If you're taking medication known to cause gynecomastia, ask your doctor if there are other choices.

Most effective Homeopathic Treatment of Male Gynecomastia

1. R-19 (Reckeweg) – 10 Drops 3 times with 1 Spoon of Water

2. Conium Mac -200 CH – 2 Drops 3 times

3. Thuja – 200 Ch – 200 CH – 2 Drops Morning

4. Kali Iodum 30 CH – 2 Drops 3 times

Infertility Involving Testicular Disease

A. Testicular Disease

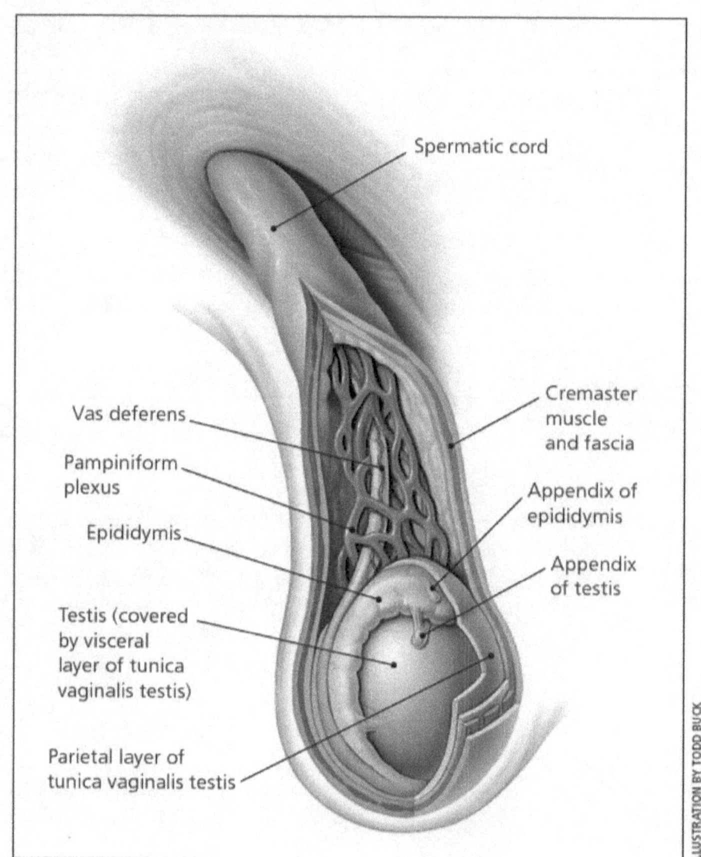

They may be rare, but testicular diseases can be life-threatening. Here's how to recognize them.

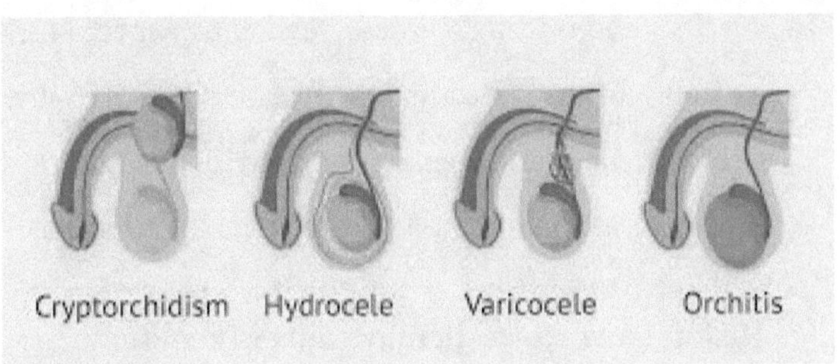

A-1. Why should I care about testicular disease?

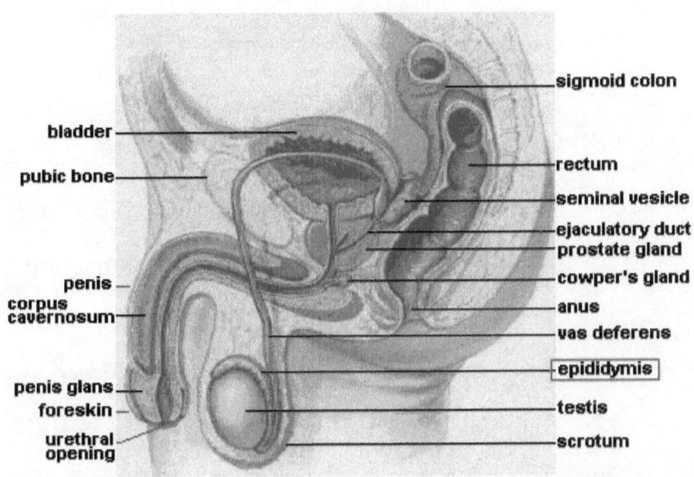

Happily, significant testicular disease is uncommon and usually not serious. But if you have any testicular pain or a change in your testicles -- such as a lump or firmness -- call your doctor. Even if you're embarrassed, delaying an evaluation is not worth the risk.

As you might guess, testicular cancer is the most serious form of testicular disease. It's also the most common cancer in men ages 18 to 35, accounting for 1% of cancer in men in the U.S. It is usually curable.

Risk factors for testicular cancer include:

- ➢ Previous history of testicular cancer
- ➢ Undescended testicle as a child
- ➢ A close relative with testicular cancer

- ➢ More common than testicular cancer is epididymitis, which is inflammation of the epididymis, a tubular structure next to the testicle where sperm mature. About 600,000 men get it each year, most commonly between ages 19 and 35. Unprotected sex or having multiple sex partners increases the risk of infectious epididymitis.
- ➢ As many as one out of every five men has varicocele, which refers to swollen and dilated

veins above the testicles (not unlike varicose veins), a condition that is usually benign.

> Hydroceles, which come from increased fluid around the testicle, also pose little risk.

A-2. What is testicular disease?

Testicular disease can take a variety of forms:

Testicular cancer.

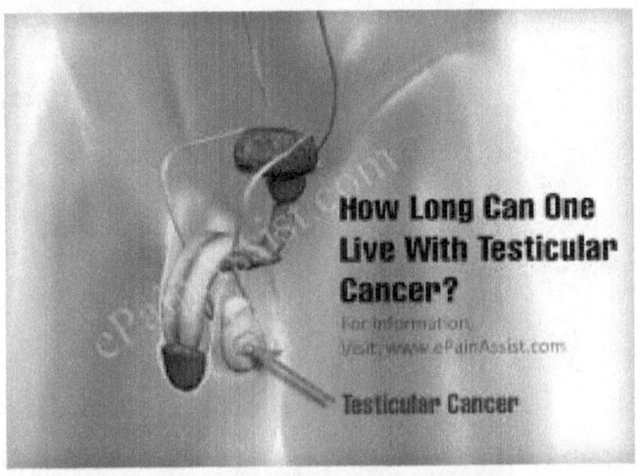

Like any cancer, testicular cancer happens when cells in the testicle develop mutations that cause them to "misbehave." The cells may multiply recklessly and invade areas where they don't belong. In testicular cancer, this process usually creates a slow-growing painless lump or firmness in one testicle. In most cases, the man himself discovers it at an early stage. If a man gets medical attention early on, testicular cancer is almost always curable.

Testicular torsion.

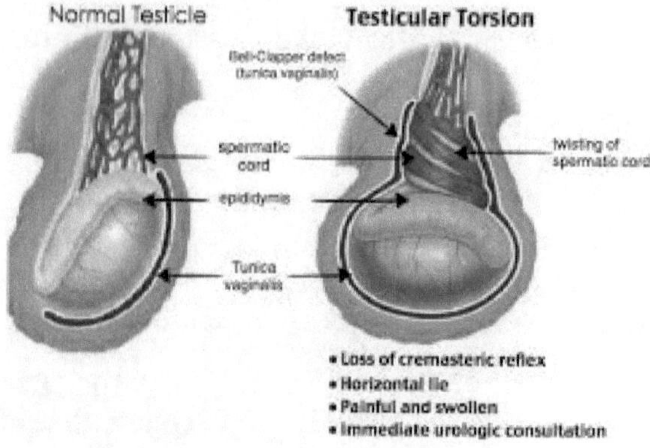

Torsion means twisting and for a testicle, that's not a good thing. When testicular torsion occurs, twisting kinks like a garden hose and blocks the blood vessels to one testicle. Certain men have a developmental problem that makes them susceptible to testicular torsion. Although testicular torsion is rare, it is an emergency. Sudden testicular pain demands an immediate trip to the emergency room. If treatment is delayed, the testicle can die. Torsion is most common during puberty - between ages 10 and 15 -- so it's important to let young teens know that any pain should be reported, even if they are embarrassed to say so.

Epididymitis.

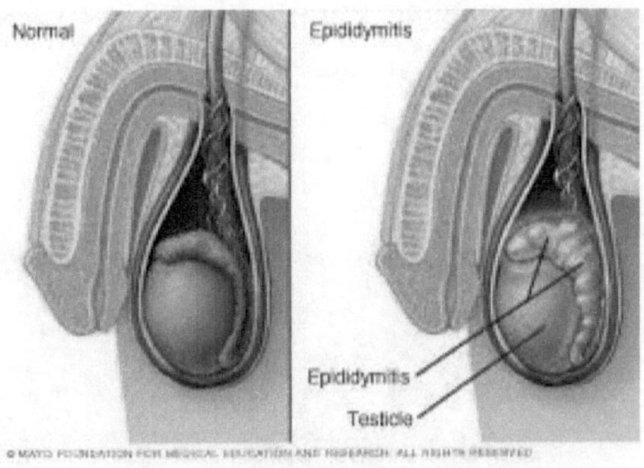

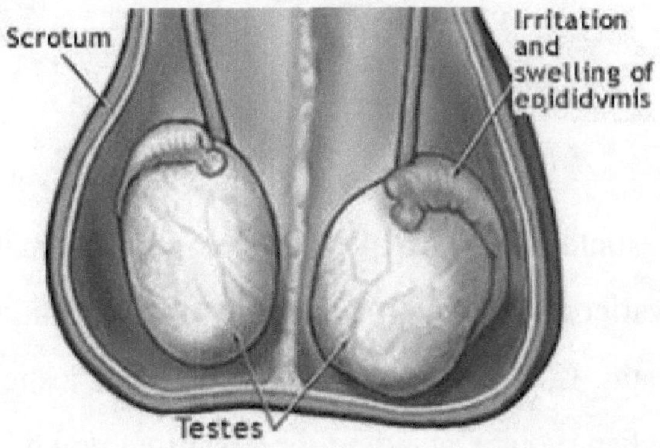

The epididymis is a long, coiled tube that sits alongside the testicle. Its job is to store sperm while they mature. Epididymitis occurs when the epididymis become inflamed or infected. Sometimes, this is a sexually transmitted infection. More often, epididymitis comes from injury, a buildup of pressure such as after a vasectomy, or from urine backwashing into the tubules during heavy lifting or straining. Epididymitis can cause symptoms ranging from mild irritation to severe testicle pain, swelling, and fever.

Varicocele.

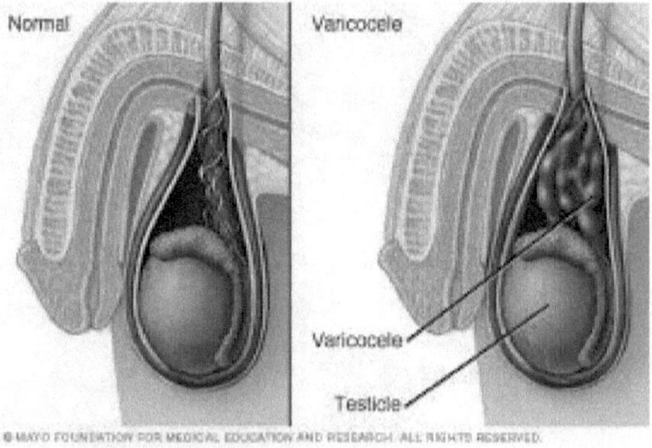

Varicocele is a dilation of the veins above the testicle and is usually harmless. Occasionally, however, varicoceles can impair fertility or cause mild to moderate pain. If you have a bulge above your testicle, especially when you're standing or "bearing down," you should have a doctor examine you.

Hydrocele.

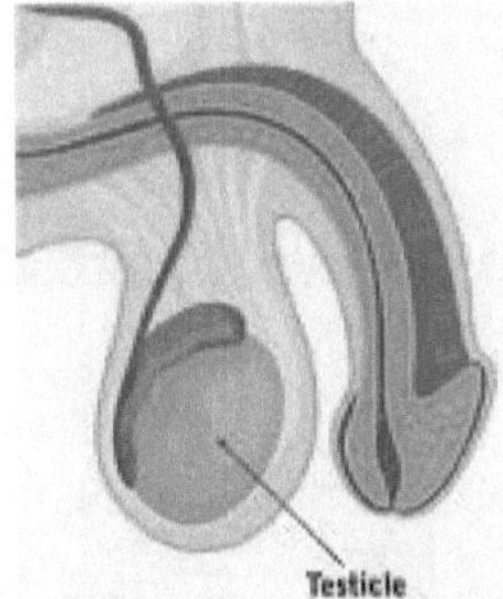

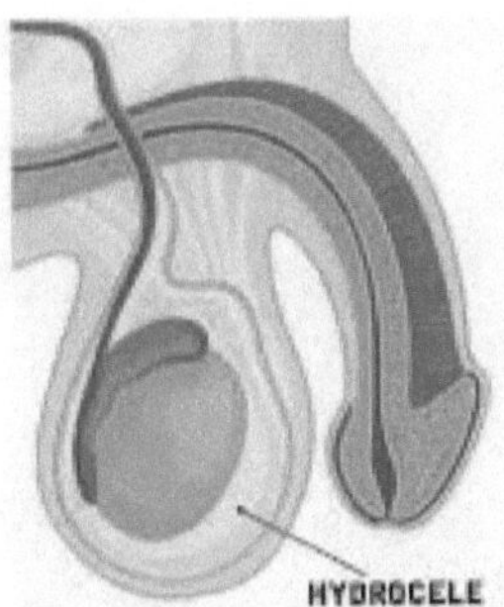

Hydrocele refers to a fluid collection surrounding the testicle and is usually benign. But if it is large enough, it can cause pain or pressure. Though men can develop a hydrocele after injury, the majority of men with hydroceles have no obvious trauma or known cause.

Orchitis.

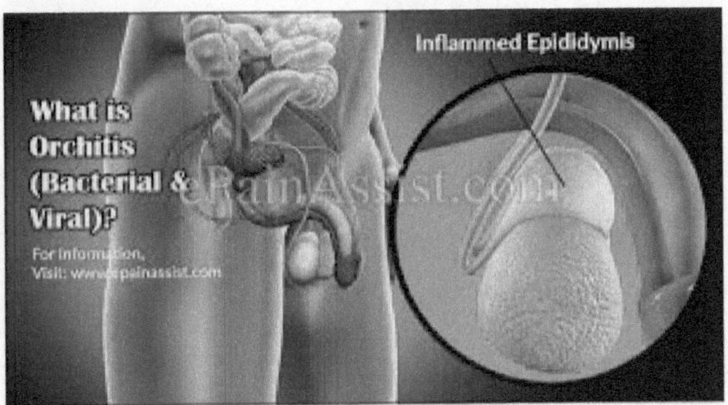

Orchitis is an inflammation of one or both testicles caused by infection or the mumps. It can also be caused by STDs like gonorrhea and chlamydia.

A-3. What can I do to prevent testicular disease?

There is no proven way to prevent testicular cancer. This is why early detection is so important. Experts recommend that all young men perform a testicular self-exam monthly. There also is no recommended method to prevent varicoceles, hydroceles, or testicular torsion.

Epididymitis can sometimes be prevented by practicing safe sex and avoiding heavy lifting or straining with a full bladder.

Varicoceles usually don't require treatment. But for men with varicoceles and impaired fertility, microsurgery to tie off the dilated veins of the varicocele is effective. Varicoceles can also be corrected without surgery by injecting a tiny coil into the abnormal veins.

If a hydrocele is very large or causing pain, surgery can usually correct it. Injecting a special material through the scrotal wall can sometimes fix hydroceles without surgery.

A- 4. What else do I need to know about testicular disease?

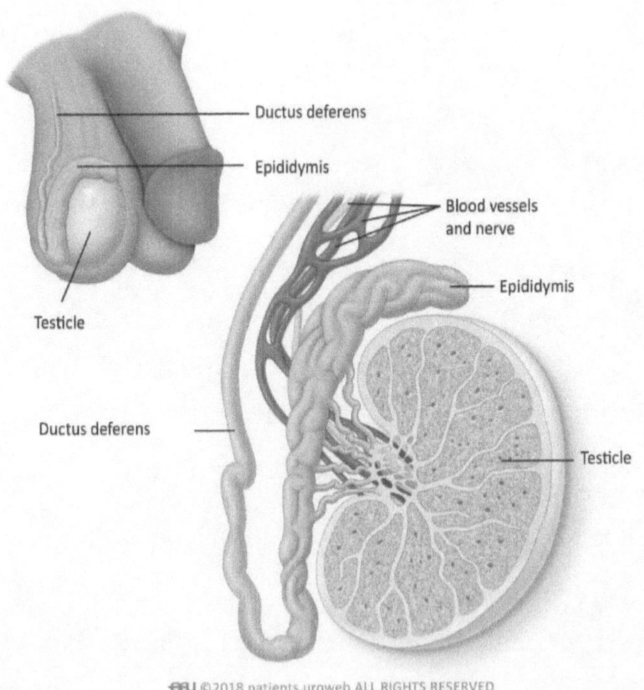

Hernias are sometimes mistaken for testicular disease. When a lower part of the abdominal wall muscles are weak, part of the intestine can bulge through it. When the intestine pushes into the scrotum, it's called an inguinal hernia -- although the scrotum swells, and it can appear to be a testicular problem. The solution is surgery to fix the weak part of the abdominal wall.

B. Testicular Cancer

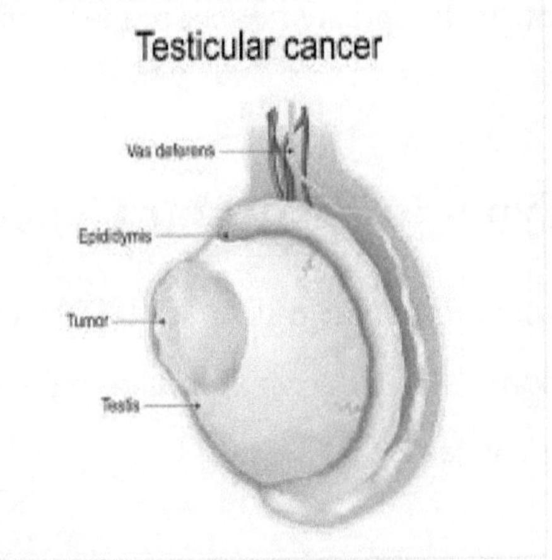

B-1. What Is It?

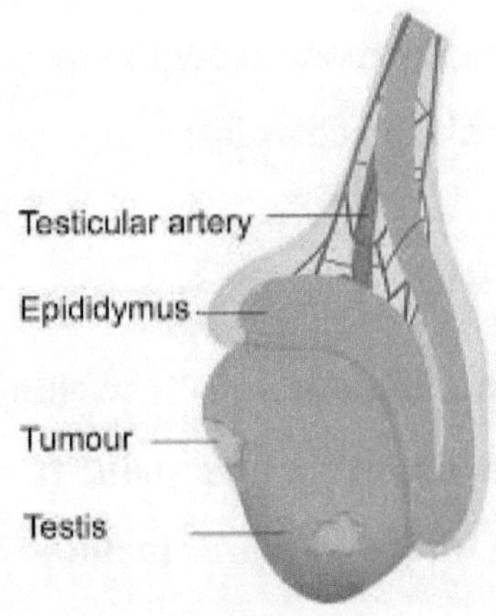

Testicles -- the male sex organs that hang in the scrotum, just below the penis -- make sperm and the hormone testosterone. Like most other parts of your body, they can get cancer. It's rare compared with other cancers, but it's the most common one in men ages 15 to 35. Even if it spreads outside the testicle, it's very treatable.

B-2. Types of Testicular Cancer

Most testicular cancer starts in germ cells, which make sperm. There are two main types of germ cell testicular cancer:

Non-seminomas tend to happen in younger men and spread quickly.

Older men are more likely to have seminomas -- these typically don't spread as fast as non-seminomas.

B-3. Symptoms

The most common sign is swelling or a lump in a testicle that doesn't cause pain. It may be pea-sized or larger. Other symptoms include:

> - Changes in how a testicle feels -- it may feel firmer or have a different texture
> - A feeling of heaviness or weight in the scrotum

> ➢ Pain, discomfort, or a dull ache in the testicles, scrotum, lower belly, or groin
> ➢ Sudden buildup of fluid in the scrotum

B-4. When to See Your Doctor

If you have pain, swelling, or a lump in one of your testicles, go see your doctor. Don't put it off more than 2 weeks. If it is cancer, early treatment can make you more likely to be cured. If you wait to go to your doctor, that gives the cancer time to spread to other parts of your body.

B-5. What Causes It?

Doctors don't know what causes testicular cancer. They know it starts like other types, when certain cells begin to grow out of control and form a tumor. But researchers are trying to figure out what triggers that. Still, some things are known to boost your odds of having it.

B-6. Who Gets It?

> ＋ Age, race, and other conditions can make you more likely to get testicular cancer:

- Infants and older males can get it, but it mostly affects men 15 to 35.
- White males get it more than others.
- Conditions that affect how testicles develop can raise your chances. One example is Klinefelter syndrome, a genetic condition that can make you more likely to have an undescended testicle.

B-7. An Undescended Testicle

Before birth, the testicles develop in a baby's belly. They usually drop into the scrotum by the time he's born or at least by age 1. But sometimes, one (or both) don't drop -- this is an undescended testicle. Men who had this problem are more likely to get testicular cancer, even if they had surgery to correct it. Surgery still helps, though -- testicles are easier to check when they're in the scrotum.

B-8. Personal or Family History

You're more likely to get it if a close relative, like your father or brother, has it. If that's the case, do self-exams to check for lumps about once a month. And if you had cancer in one testicle, you have higher odds of getting it in the other one. Make sure to go to all your scheduled follow-ups.

B-9. How It's Diagnosed: Blood Tests

In many cases, men find a lump on their own or their doctor finds one during a routine exam. If your doctor thinks it might be cancer, he may recommend a blood test to look for markers -- things in your blood, like proteins or hormones that can be higher if you have a tumor.

B-10. How It's Diagnosed: Ultrasound and Surgery

With other types of cancer, doctors often test a tumor sample for cancer. But they don't do that for testicular cancer, because that can damage a testicle and cause the cancer to spread. Instead, your doctor probably will do an ultrasound, which makes images of your scrotum and testicles. If it looks like you have cancer, you may have surgery to remove the testicle and have it tested. This will tell if it's cancer and what kind it is.

B-11. Staging Tests

If you're diagnosed with testicular cancer, you'll need more tests to see where it might have spread. It helps your doctor decide the kind of treatment you'll need. You'll typically have:

A computerized tomography (CT) scan, which takes X-rays from several angles and puts them together to make detailed images of your belly, chest, and pelvis

Blood tests to see if markers are still in your blood after your testicle has been removed

B-12. Stages

The stage of your cancer will be based on the size of the tumor and how far it's spread:

Stage I: The cancer is only in your testicle and hasn't spread anywhere else.

Stage II: The cancer has spread to lymph nodes in your belly.

Stage III: The cancer has spread to other parts of your body, like your lungs, liver, bones, or brain.

B-13. Self-Exams

Your doctor may recommend that you check for lumps each month, especially if you're more likely to get testicular cancer. To do these exams:

- Shower or bathe first so the scrotum is loose.
- Stand in front of a mirror to look for swelling in the scrotum.
- Hold your testicle between your thumbs and fingers and roll it gently.
- Feel for lumps or changes in texture.

C. Prostate Cancer?

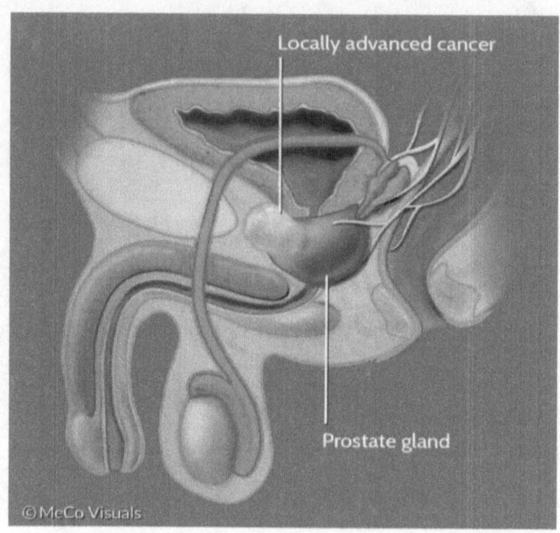

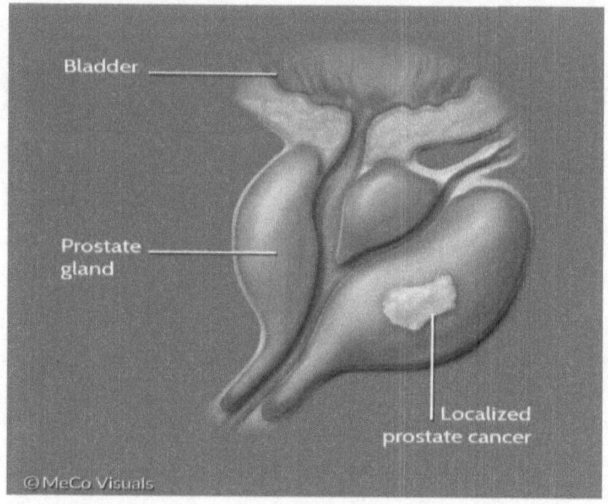

Prostate cancer develops in a man's prostate, the walnut-sized gland just below the bladder that produces some of the fluid in semen. It's the most common cancer in men after skin cancer. Prostate cancer often grows very slowly and may not cause significant harm. But some types are more aggressive and can spread quickly without treatment.

C-1. Symptoms of Prostate Cancer

- In the early stages, men may have no symptoms. Later, symptoms can include:
- Frequent urination, especially at night
- Difficulty starting or stopping urination
- Weak or interrupted urinary stream
- Painful or burning sensation during urination or ejaculation
- Blood in urine or semen
- Advanced cancer can cause deep pain in the lower back, hips, or upper thighs.

C-2. Enlarged Prostate or Prostate Cancer?

The prostate can grow larger as men age, sometimes pressing on the bladder or urethra and causing symptoms similar to prostate cancer. This is called benign prostatic hyperplasia (BPH). It's not cancer and can be treated if symptoms become bothersome. A third problem that can cause urinary symptoms is prostatitis. This inflammation or infection may also cause a fever and in many cases is treated with medication.

C-3. Risk Factors You Can't Control

Growing older is the greatest risk factor for prostate cancer, particularly after age 50. After age 70, studies suggest that anywhere from 31% to 83% of men have some form of prostate cancer, though there may be no outward symptoms. Family history increases a man's risk: having a father or brother with prostate cancer more than doubles the risk. African-American men and Caribbean men of African descent are at high risk and have the highest rate of prostate cancer in the world.

C-4. Risk Factors You Can Control

Diet seems to play a role in the development of prostate cancer, which is much more common in countries where meat and high-fat dairy are mainstays. The reason for this link is unclear. Dietary fat, particularly animal fat from red meat, may boost male hormone levels. And this may fuel the growth of cancerous prostate cells. A diet too low in fruits and vegetables may also play a role.

C-5. Myths About Prostate Cancer

Here are some things that will not cause prostate cancer: Too much sex, a vasectomy, and masturbation. If you have an enlarged prostate (BPH), that does not mean you are at greater risk of developing prostate cancer. Researchers are still studying whether alcohol use, STDs, or prostatitis play a role in the development of prostate cancer.

C-6. Can Prostate Cancer Be Found Early?

*   Screening tests are available to find prostate cancer early, but government guidelines don't call for routine testing in men at any age. The tests may find cancers that are so slow-growing that medical treatments would offer no benefit. And the treatments themselves can have serious side effects. The American Cancer

Society advises men to talk with a doctor about screening tests, beginning at:

*   Age 50 for average-risk men who expect to live at least 10 more years

*   Age 45 for men at high risk; this includes African-Americans and those with a father, brother, or son diagnosed before age 65

*   Age 40 for men with more than one first-degree relative diagnosed at an early age

*   The U.S. Preventive Services Task Force (USPSTF) says that testing may be appropriate for some men age 55 – 69. They recommend that men talk to their doctor to discuss the potential risks and benefits of being tested.

C-7. Screening: DRE and PSA

Your doctor may initially do a digital rectal exam (DRE) to feel for bumps or hard spots on the prostate. After a discussion with your doctor, a blood test can be used to measure prostate-specific antigen (PSA), a protein produced by prostate cells. An elevated level may indicate a higher chance that you have cancer, but you can have a high level and still be cancer-free. It is also possible to have a normal PSA and have prostate cancer.

C-8. PSA Test Results

*   A normal PSA level is considered to be under 4 nanograms per milliliter (ng/mL) of blood, while a PSA above 10 suggests a high risk of cancer. But there are many exceptions:

*   Men can have prostate cancer with a PSA less than 4.

*   A prostate that is inflamed (prostatitis) or enlarged (BPH) can boost PSA levels, yet further testing may show no evidence of cancer.

*   Some BPH drugs can lower PSA levels, despite the presence of prostate cancer, called a false negative.

*   If either a PSA or DRE test are abnormal, your doctor will likely order other tests.

C-9. Prostate Cancer Biopsy

If a physical exam or PSA test suggests a problem, your doctor may recommend a biopsy. A needle is inserted either through the rectum wall or the skin between the rectum and scrotum. Multiple small tissue samples are removed and examined under a microscope. A biopsy is the best way to detect cancer and predict whether it is slow-growing or aggressive.

C-10. Biopsy and Gleason Score

A pathologist looks for cell abnormalities and "grades" the tissue sample from 1 to 5. The sum of two Gleason grades is the Gleason score. These scores help determine the chances of the cancer spreading. Gleason grades of 1 and 2 are not usually given in biopsies, so 6 is typically the lowest score for a prostate cancer. Cancer with Gleason scores of 8 to 10 is called high-grade, and can grow and spread more quickly. Gleason scores help guide the type of treatment your doctor will recommend.

C-11. Prostate Cancer Imaging

Some men may need additional tests to see if the cancer has spread beyond the prostate. These can include ultrasound, a CT scan, or an MRI scan (seen here). A radionuclide bone scan traces an injection of low-level radioactive material to help detect cancer that has spread to the bone.

In the MRI scan shown here, the tumor is the green, kidney-shaped mass in the center, next to the prostate gland (in pink).

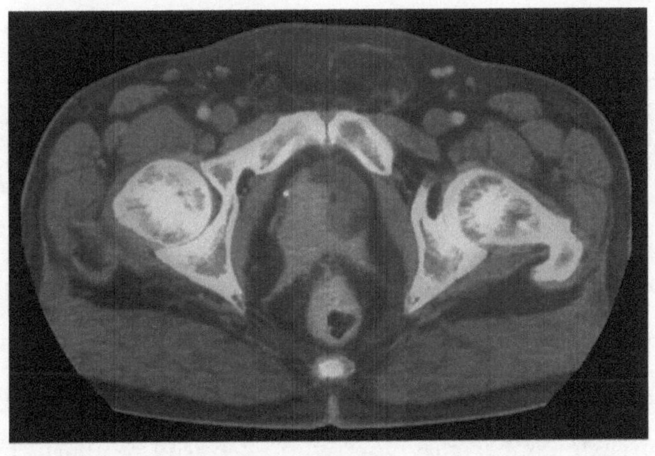

C-12. Prostate Cancer Staging

Staging is used to describe how far prostate cancer has spread (metastasized) and to help determine the best treatment.

Stage I: Cancer is small and still within the prostate.

Stage II: Cancer is more advanced, but still confined to the prostate.

Stage III: Cancer is a high grade or it has spread beyond the outer part of the prostate or into nearby tissues such as seminal vesicles, the bladder, or rectum.

Stage IV: Cancer has spread to lymph nodes or distant organs such as bones or lungs.

C-13. Hope for Advanced Cancer

Your doctor will continue to monitor your PSA levels and may perform other tests after treatment for prostate cancer. If it recurs or spreads to other parts of the body, additional treatment may be recommended. Lifestyle choices may matter, too. One study found that prostate cancer survivors who exercised regularly had a lower risk of dying, for example.

C-14. Food for Health

A cancer-conscious diet may be the best choice for survivors who want to bolster their health and those hoping to lower their risk. That means:

> ➤ Five or more fruits and veggies a day
> ➤ Whole grains instead of white flour or white rice
> ➤ Limit high-fat meat
> ➤ Limit or eliminate processed meat (hot dogs, cold cuts, bacon)
> ➤ Limit alcohol to 1-2 drinks per day (if you drink)
> ➤ Studies found mixed results on lycopene, an antioxidant found in tomatoes.

C-15. Supplements: Buyer Beware

Be wary of supplements that are marketed to prevent prostate cancer. Some herbal substances can interfere with PSA levels. Study results have been mixed on the impact that taking selenium and vitamin E have on the risk of prostate cancer. Be sure to tell your doctor if you are taking vitamins or supplements

C-16. (Most effective Homeopathic medicine for Prostate Cancer)

Sabal serrulata Q	15 Drops, 3 Times, with ½ Cup of Water
Thuja 200	4 Drops, Every day Morning
Chimaphila umbellata Q	15 Drops, 3 Times, with ½ Cup of Water
Cannabis indica 30	2 Drops, 2 Times,
Cantharis 200	2 Drops, 2 Times,
Conium Mac 1M	4 Drops, Once in a Week
Carcinosium **200**	4 Drops, Once in a Week

D. All about BPH?

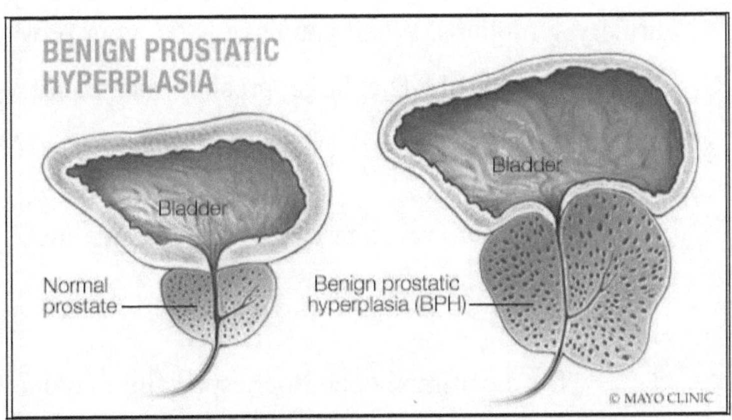

D-1. What Is BPH?

*   You can do a lot to take care of yourself and give your body what it needs. Still, as you get older, your body changes in ways you can't always control. For most men, one of those changes is that the prostate gets bigger.

*   It's a natural part of aging, but at some point, it can lead to a condition called BPH, or benign prostatic hyperplasia.

*   Your prostate surrounds part of your urethra, the tube that carries urine and semen out of your penis. When

you have BPH, your prostate is larger than usual, which squeezes the urethra. This can cause your pee stream to be weak, waking you up a lot at night to go to the bathroom along. it also could lead to other bothersome urinary symptoms. When you have BPH, your prostate is larger than usual. The large prostate can squeeze the urethra.

*   BPH isn't prostate cancer and doesn't make you more likely to get it.

*   It's a common condition, especially in older men, and there are a lot of treatments for it, from lifestyle changes to medication to surgery. Your doctor can help you choose the best care based on your age, health, and how the condition affects you.

D-2. What Causes BPH?

*   Doctors aren't sure exactly what makes this happen. Some think it may have to do with normal hormonal changes as you age, but it's not clear.

*   Early in puberty, your prostate actually doubles in size. Later in life, around age 25, it starts to grow

again. For most men, this growth happens for the rest of their lives. For some, it causes BPH.

D-3. Symptoms

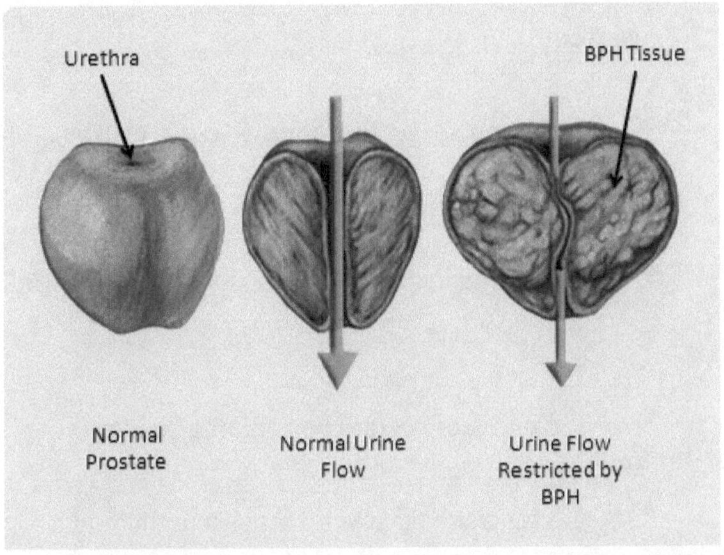

*   As the prostate gets larger, it starts to pinch the urethra. This causes symptoms that affect your urine flow, such as:

*   Dribbling when you finish

*   A hard time getting started

*   A weak stream, or you pee in stops and starts

*   When your urethra is squeezed, it also means your bladder has to work harder to push urine out. Over time, the bladder muscles get weak, which makes it harder for it to empty. This can lead to:

*   Feeling like you still have to pee even after you just went

*   Having to go too often -- eight or more times a day

*   Incontinence (when you don't have control over when you pee)

*   An urgent need to pee, all of a sudden

*   You wake up several times a night to pee

*   A larger prostate doesn't mean you'll have more or worse symptoms. It's different for each person. In fact, some men with very large prostates have few, if any, issues.

D-4. Diagnosis and Tests

Your doctor will first talk to you about your personal and family medical history. You might also fill out a survey, answering questions about your symptoms and how they affect you daily.

Next, your doctor will do a physical exam. This may include a digital rectal exam. During this, he puts on a glove and gently inserts one finger into your rectum to check the size and shape of your prostate.

D-5. Basic tests:

Your doctor may start with one or more of these:

> Blood tests to check for kidney problems
> Urine tests to look for infection or other problems that could be causing your symptoms
> PSA (prostate-specific antigen) blood test. High PSA levels may be a sign of a larger-than-usual prostate. A doctor can also order it as screening for prostate cancer.

D-6. Advanced tests:

Based on the results of those tests, your doctor may order additional tests to rule out other problems or to see more clearly what's happening. These might include:

- Different types of ultrasound to measure your prostate and see if it looks healthy.
- A bladder ultrasound to see how well you empty your bladder.
- Biopsy to rule out cancer.
- Urine flow test to measure how strong your stream is and how much pee you make.
- Urodynamics testing to evaluate your bladder function.
- Cystourethroscopy is a procedure using a camera to examine the inside of the prostate, urethra and bladder.

D-7. Lifestyle changes:

You may want to start with things you can control. For example, you can:

- ✓ Do exercises to strengthen your pelvic floor muscles
- ✓ Lower the amount of fluids you drink, especially before you go out or go to bed
- ✓ Drink less caffeine and alcohol

D-8. Procedures:

If lifestyle changes and medications don't work, your doctor has a number of ways to remove part or all of your prostate. Many of these are called "minimally invasive," meaning they're easier on you than regular surgery. They use probes or scopes and don't require large cuts in your body.

*   Examples of a minimally invasive procedures are TUMT, TUNA, or Rezūm which use a varied form of energy to destroy part of the prostate.

*   Other, more involved surgical procedures include:

*   Laser therapy to remove part of your prostate

*   Transurethral resection of the prostate, or TURP, in which the doctor uses a scope and cuts out pieces of the gland with a wire loop

*   Transurethral incision of the prostate or TUIP, in which a few small cuts are made in the prostate to reduce the gland's pressure on the urethra.

*   UroLift system is a permanently placed device used to lift and hold the enlarged prostate tissue out of the way, so it no longer blocks the urethra

*   In some cases, your doctor may also suggest a traditional, open surgery or a robotic procedure to remove your prostate.

D-9. Any Complications?

With any BPH surgery, there may be side effects or complications such as bleeding, narrowing of the urine tube also known as urethral stricture, urinary incontinence or leakage, erectile dysfunction, and retrograde ejaculation.

*   BPH doesn't lead to prostate cancer or make you more likely to get it.

*   It rarely leads to other conditions, but it can, and a couple of them are serious. For example, BPH can lead to kidney damage or, worst-case, cause a problem where you can't pee at all.

It may also cause:

- Bladder damage
- Bladder stones
- Urinary tract infections
- Blood in your urine

D.10. What Are the Symptoms of BPH?

*   As they age, some men may notice that they have trouble peeing. You might find it hard to start going, or perhaps the stream starts and stops several times.

*   These are just two possible signs of benign prostatic hyperplasia, called BPH, which is an enlarged prostate.

This gland, which grows during early puberty and then again around age 25, becomes enlarged in many men. It can pinch your urethra, the tube that carries urine from your bladder through your penis. Your bladder walls may also grow thicker.

This is the most common prostate problem in men 50 and older. It's good to know the symptoms of BPH because you might want to talk with your doctor.

D-11. What Should I Watch Out For?

Symptoms of BPH fall into 2 categories. Those caused by pressure on your urethra are called obstructive. The others start in your bladder.

Some of the obstructive symptoms include:

> ➢ Trouble starting to urinate
> ➢ You have to strain or push when you pee
> ➢ The stream is weak
> ➢ You have to stop and restart several times
> ➢ Pee dribbles out at the end

If BPH causes changes in your bladder, it may include these signs:

- You suddenly feel a strong need to urinate. Doctors call this "urgency."

- You have to pee more than 8 times a day. This is called "frequency."

- Even after you go, you feel as though your bladder is not empty.

- You wake up often in the night to relieve yourself. This is called "nocturia."

D-12. Complications

* If you don't get treatment for prostate problems, your bladder can become irritated because urine is backing up rather than being released.

* Your symptoms may start to cause more issues in your day-to-day life. For instance, it may be tough for you to control your bladder. You might wet the bed at night or not be able to get to the bathroom quickly enough when the urgent need to go strikes.

* You also could develop an infection in your urinary tract or get bladder stones.

* Some symptoms of BPH are not as common, and they could signal that your condition is more complicated or advanced. Those signs include:

*   Burning or pain when you pee

*   Blood in your urine

 You can't go at all because your urethra is blocked. Get emergency treatment right away if this happens.

D-13. When Should I Call a Doctor?

*   Your symptoms may not bother you too much. But it's important to talk over any urinary problems with your doctor.

*   It's hard to predict how BPH will play out, and you can't assume that the problem will get better on its own. Your doctor also will want to rule out things that cause similar problems.

Some symptoms need quick medical attention. If you have any of these, call your doctor right away or head to an emergency room:

- ✓ You can't urinate at all.
- ✓ You have to pee frequently, it's painful, and you have fever and chills.
- ✓ You have blood in your urine.

✓ You feel a great deal of pain in your lower belly and urinary tract.

D-14. What Tests Do I Need for BPH?

* Benign prostatic hyperplasia, or BPH, is an enlarged prostate gland. Its symptoms can look like prostate cancer, but it's not. BPH symptoms can also be hard to tell apart from urinary tract infections and bladder or kidney problems.

* Your doctor can do tests like a digital rectal exam and a biopsy to know for sure whether you have BPH.

* Once you have a diagnosis, treatments can help you avoid complications such as urinary tract infections or damage to the bladder or kidneys.

D-15. BPH Questions

* The American Urological Association has a ratings system to rate how severe your symptoms are. It's called the "BPH Symptom Score Index."

It includes 7 questions about what's been happening with you over the past month. They are:

- How often have you felt like you weren't able to fully empty your bladder when you finished peeing?
- How often have you had to go again less than 2 hours after you last finished?
- How often have you stopped and started while peeing?
- How often have you found it hard to wait to go?
- How often have you had a weak stream?
- How often have you had to push or strain to start urinating?
- How many times do you have to get up and use the bathroom during the night?

Each question is assigned points from 0 (none at all) to 5 (almost always). Your score will show whether your BPH is mild or severe and guide your treatment.

D-16. Diagnosis

You can see your usual doctor for a diagnosis, or you can visit a urologist, who is a specialist in diseases of the urinary tract and male reproductive system. This will likely involve the following:

Medical history:

He will first ask you questions about your health and any medicines you take.

General physical:

Then you'll have a physical exam. The doctor will feel your belly and groin areas to check for any lumps.

Digital rectal exam:

This is a way for your doctor to feel if your prostate is enlarged. The prostate is right next to your rectum.

First, you'll bend over the exam table or you might lie on your side with your knees pulled up to your chest. Your doctor will gently slide a gloved, lubricated finger into your rectum to feel your prostate. He will feel for any growths or lumps.

You might feel the need to pee or a little discomfort, but the exam should be quick.

D-17. Other Tests

These tests can look for other causes of BPH symptoms, such as a urinary tract infection, a bladder problem, or prostate cancer.

Urine test.

For this, you'll pee into a cup. A treated piece of paper placed into your urine can show whether you have an infection. It might also be checked for small traces of blood that could signal bladder cancer or other conditions.

Blood test.

This can check your levels of two chemical waste products: creatinine and blood urea nitrogen. High levels of these might mean your kidneys aren't working as well as they should.

PSA test.

This checks for levels of what's called prostate specific antigen, or PSA, in your blood. PSA is a protein your prostate makes. Both BPH and prostate cancer can raise your PSA level. This test alone can't confirm that you have BPH. You will need other tests, too. If your level is high and your doctor suspects cancer, you'll likely have a prostate biopsy.

Urodynamic tests.

This group of tests checks how well you hold and release urine in your bladder and your urethra, which is the narrow tube in your penis through which pee and semen flow. You might get these tests at your doctor's office or at a hospital.

A post-void residual measurement

Checks how much urine is left in your bladder after you go to the bathroom. First you will be asked to pee. Then the doctor will place a thin tube called a catheter into your urethra. The tube will be threaded into your bladder to remove any urine that's left inside. That leftover liquid is measured. It can also be checked with an office ultrasound or bladder scanner. Cold jelly is placed over the bladder and the ultrasound measures the left over urine.

Uroflowmetry

measures how fast you release urine. This is called your flow rate. During the test, you'll pee into a special toilet or container. A slow flow might mean you have weak bladder muscles or a blockage in your urinary tract.

Urodynamic pressure

uses a meter to find out how much pressure needs to be on your bladder for you to pee. It also tests your flow rate. This test can show whether an enlarged prostate is blocking the flow out of your bladder.

Cystoscopy.

This test lets the doctor see inside your urethra and bladder. You will first get medicine so you don't feel pain. You might be given something so you aren't awake during the test.

The doctor will insert a tube called a cystoscope through your urethra into your bladder. The tube has a lens on one end that lets him look for problems inside your urinary tract.

ultrasound.

An ultrasound uses sound waves to make a picture of your prostate gland. It can show whether it is enlarged or you have a tumor. You can have this test at your doctor's office or a hospital.

Transrectal

A technician will insert a thin device called a transducer into your rectum. As the device moves around, it will show different parts of your prostate.

Biopsy.

For this test, you will first get medicine so you don't feel any pain. The doctor will use an ultrasound, CT, or MRI scan to see your prostate gland. He will then use a needle to take a piece of tissue. The sample will be sent to a lab where a technician will look at it under a microscope to see whether it is cancerous.

Talk to your doctor about your test results. Make sure you understand what they mean and how they will affect your treatment.

D-18. Can I Prevent BPH?

Men with BPH have a larger-than-normal prostate. Some 9 in 10 men will have it by the time they're in their 80s. Even with those chances, you still might ask: Are there things I can do to prevent it?

The short answer is no. For most men, your prostate's just going to grow, and it might lead to benign prostatic hyperplasia, as it's formally known.

But it still helps to know when you'd want to see your doctor, what makes you more likely to get it, and how you can keep the symptoms at bay.

D-19. When Should I See a Doctor?

Growth of this gland, which is just below the bladder, is typical. But problems when you pee aren't. Even if you don't think it's a big deal, it's worth getting checked out if you have common BPH symptoms, such as:

➢ Dribbling when you finish peeing

➢ A hard time starting a stream

➢ Having to pee a lot -- 8 or more times a day

➢ Waking up several times a night to pee

➢ A weak urine stream or you pee in stops and starts

Some problems with urine flow can be more serious. See your doctor or go to the emergency room right away if you:

✓ Can't pee at all

✓ Feel intense pain or discomfort in your lower belly

✓ Have blood in your pee

✓ Keep needing to pee right away, it hurts to pee, and you have fever and chills

D-20. Who's More Likely to Get BPH?

You may have a greater chance of an enlarged prostate based on your:

Age. BPH is more common the older you get and doesn't usually affect men younger than 40.

Family history. If your dad or your brothers have the condition, you have a higher chance of getting it, too.

Ethnicity. This affects black and white men more often than Asian men. Black men may get symptoms at a younger age.

Some health conditions can also raise the odds you'll get BPH, such as:

- Diabetes, heart disease, and problems with blood flow
- Erectile dysfunction, Obesity
- If you use beta blockers -- a type of medication used to treat conditions such as high blood pressure and migraines -- you may be more likely to get BPH.

D-21. Can Lifestyle Changes Help?

Lifestyle changes can't prevent BPH, but they may still be good for your prostate. For starters, exercise and a heart-healthy diet can help manage your weight, which is great for your prostate. Exercise also helps your bladder empty at a normal rate.

To control symptoms, it may help to:

- ➢ Avoid or limit how you use decongestants and antihistamines during cold s and allergy outbreaks as they tighten the muscles that control urine flow and make it harder to pee
- ➢ Do exercises to strengthen your pelvic floor muscles
- ➢ Limit how much caffeine and alcohol you take in; they make you pee more and can irritate your bladder
- ➢ Lower the amount of fluids you drink, especially before you go out or go to bed.
- ➢ Pee when you first feel the urge because it's easier on your bladder.

> Stay warm. Cold can make it feel more urgent to pee.

D-22.   Most effective Homeopathic medicine for BPH

A. Sabal Serrulata Q   **20 Drops, With ½ Cup of water, 3 Times a Day**

B. Mix each 3 Drops With ½ Cup of Water & take 3 Times a Day

1. **Sabal Serrulata**   **2x**   **3 Drops**
2. **Chimaphila Umbellata 3x**   **3 Drops**
3. **Conium Mac 3x**   **3 Drops**
4. **Clematis   3x**   **3 Drops**
5. **Pareira Brava 3x**   **3 Drops**
6. **Pulsatilla   3x**   **3 Drops**

E. Varicocele

E-1. What is a varicocele?

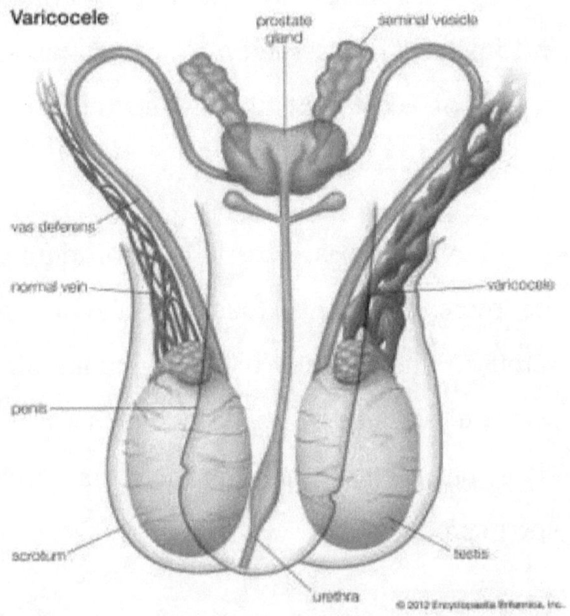

The scrotum is a skin-covered sac that holds your testicles. It also contains the arteries and veins that deliver blood to the reproductive glands. A vein abnormality in the scrotum may result in a varicocele. A varicocele is an enlargement of the veins within the scrotum. These veins are called the pampiniform plexus.

A varicocele only occurs in the scrotum and is very similar to varicose veins that can occur in the leg.

A varicocele can result in decreased sperm production and quality, which in some cases can lead to infertility. It can also shrink the testicles.

Varicoceles are common. They can be found in 15 percent of the adult male population and around 20 percent of adolescent males. They're more common in males aged 15 to 25.

Varicoceles generally form during puberty and are more commonly found on the left side of your scrotum. The anatomy of the right and left side of your scrotum isn't the same. Varicoceles can exist on both sides, but it's extremely rare. Not all varicoceles affect sperm production.

E-2. What causes a varicocele to develop?

A spermatic cord holds up each testicle. The cords also contain the veins, arteries, and nerves that support these glands. In healthy veins inside the scrotum, one-way valves move the blood from the testicles to the scrotum, and then they send it back to the heart.

Sometimes the blood doesn't move through the veins like it should and begins to pool in the vein, causing it to enlarge. A varicocele develops slowly over time.

There are no established risk factors for developing a varicocele, and the exact cause is unclear.

E-3. Recognizing the symptoms of a varicocele

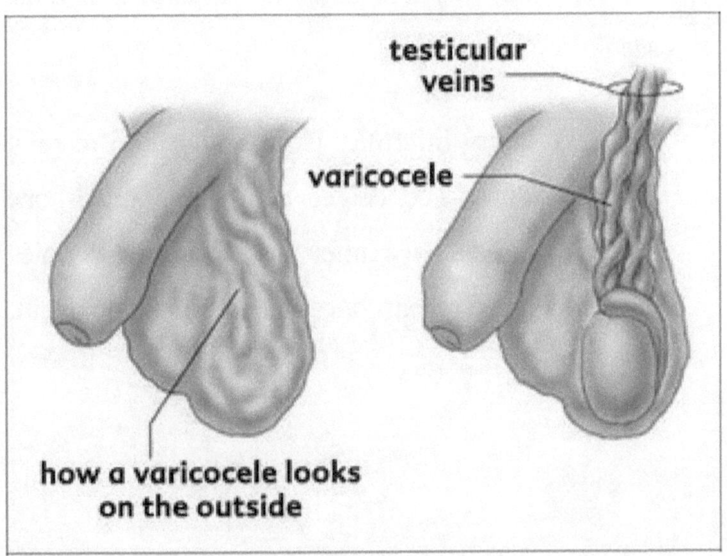

You may have no symptoms associated with a varicocele. However, you might experience:

- ✓ A lump in one of your testicles
- ✓ Swelling in your scrotum
- ✓ Visibly enlarged or twisted veins in your scrotum, which are often described as looking like a bag of worms
- ✓ A dull, recurring pain in your scrotum

E-4. Possible complications

This condition can have an effect on fertility. Varicocele is present in 35 to 44 percent of men with primary infertility and in 45 to 81 percent of men with secondary infertility.

Primary infertility is generally used to refer to a couple that hasn't conceived a child after at least one year of trying. Secondary infertility describes couples that have conceived at least once but aren't able to again.

E-5. How is a varicocele diagnosed?

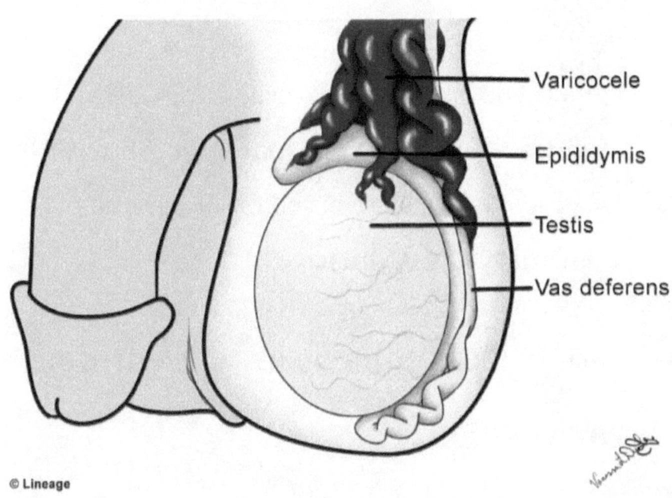

Your doctor usually diagnoses the condition after a physical exam. A varicocele can't always be felt or seen when you're lying down. Your doctor will most likely examine your testicles while you're standing up and lying down.

Your doctor may need to perform a scrotal ultrasound. This helps measure the spermatic veins and allows your doctor to get a detailed, accurate picture of the condition.

Once the varicocele is diagnosed, your doctor will classify it with one of three clinical grades. They're labeled grades 1 through 3, according to the size of the lump in your testicle. Grade 1 is the smallest and grade 3 the largest.

The size doesn't necessarily affect the overall treatment because you may not require treatment. Treatment options are based on the degree of discomfort or infertility issues you have.

E-6. Methods of treatment for varicoceles

It's not always necessary to treat a varicocele. However, you may want to consider treatment if the varicocele:

> causes pain

> causes testicular atrophy

> causes infertility

You may also want to consider treatment if you're thinking about assisted reproductive techniques.

This condition can cause problems with testicular functioning in some people. The earlier you start treatment, the better your chances of improving sperm production.

Wearing tight underwear or a jock strap can sometimes provide you with support that alleviates pain or discomfort. Additional treatment, such as varicocelectomy and varicocele embolization, might be necessary if your symptoms get worse.

E-7. Varicocele embolization

Varicocele embolization is a less invasive, same-day procedure. A small catheter is inserted into a groin or neck vein. A coil is then placed into the catheter and into the varicocele. This blocks blood from getting to the abnormal veins.

E-8. Living with a varicocele

Infertility is a common complication of a varicocele. Talk to your doctor about seeing a reproductive specialist if you and your partner are having problems getting pregnant.

E-9. Most effective Homeopathic medicine for varicoceles

Sr. No	Healing Substance	Power	Formula	Doses
1	Hamamelis	30	Mix 10 ml of each in a new Bottle	15 Drops with ½ cup of water
2	Aesculus	30		
3	Belladonna	30		
4	Calcium Fluoratum	30		
5	Carduus Marianus	200		
6	Mezereum	200		
7	Placenta (Suis)	30		
8	Pulsatilla	30		
9	Secale comutum	30		
10	Vipera Berus	200		
11	CALCAREA FLUORICA	6 X	4 (Tablets) a day	3 Times
12	Thuja	200	4 Drops morning daily	

F. Hydrocele

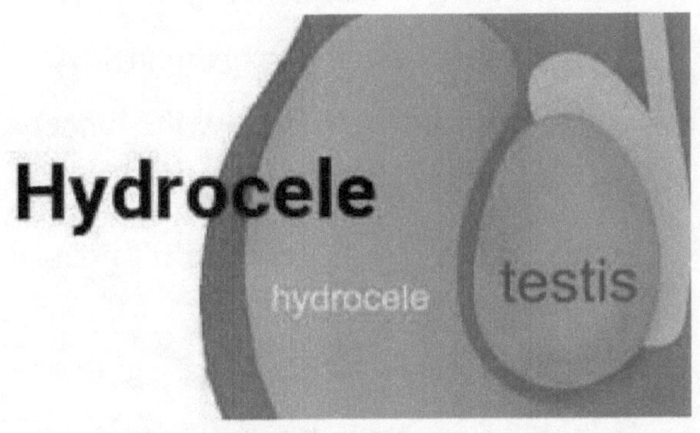

F-1. Hydrocele in Baby Boys

A hydrocele is a swelling in a boy's scrotum, the thin sac that holds his testicles. It happens when too much fluid builds up inside. The condition is most common in newborns, though older boys and men can get it, too.

It may sound or look serious, even painful, but don't worry, it won't hurt your baby. It might even go away on its own, though you should still see the doctor about it.

F-2. Causes

A hydrocele can start before your son is born. His testicles grow inside his belly and then move down into his scrotum through a short tunnel. A sac of fluid goes with each testicle. Normally, the tunnel and the sac seal off before birth, and the baby's body absorbs the fluid inside. When this process doesn't go as it should, he can get a hydrocele.

There are two types:

Noncommunicating hydrocele happens when the sac closes like normal, but the boy's body doesn't absorb the fluid inside it.

Communicating hydrocele happens when the sac doesn't seal. With this type, his scrotum may swell more over time.

Babies born prematurely are more likely to have a hydrocele.

F-3. Symptoms

A hydrocele doesn't hurt. The only symptom you'll notice is that one or both of your son's testicles look swollen. Even if he's not in pain, you should see the pediatrician to make sure he doesn't have other health problems that are causing the swelling, such as an infection, a tumor, or a hernia.

The swelling from a no communicating hydrocele doesn't change in size. A communicating hydrocele can get bigger during the day, and if you gently squeeze it, the fluid will move out of the scrotum and into his belly.

F-4. Getting a Diagnosis

When you take your son to the doctor, she'll do a physical exam. She'll check his scrotum for fluid and tenderness, and she'll shine a light through it to see if there's fluid around his testicle.

She'll also check to make sure your baby doesn't have a hernia.

Your son may also have a blood test and an ultrasound to make sure nothing else is causing the swelling.

F-6. Most effective Homeopathic medicine for varicoceles Hydrocele

Sr. No	Healing Substance	Power	Drops	No. of doses in a day
1	Rhododendron	30	2	3
2	Clematis	30	2	3
3	Graphites	30	2	Morning
4	Natrum mur	6 x	6 (Tab)	3
5	Arnica	30	2	3

G. Inflammation of the Testicle (Orchitis)

G-1. What is Orchitis?

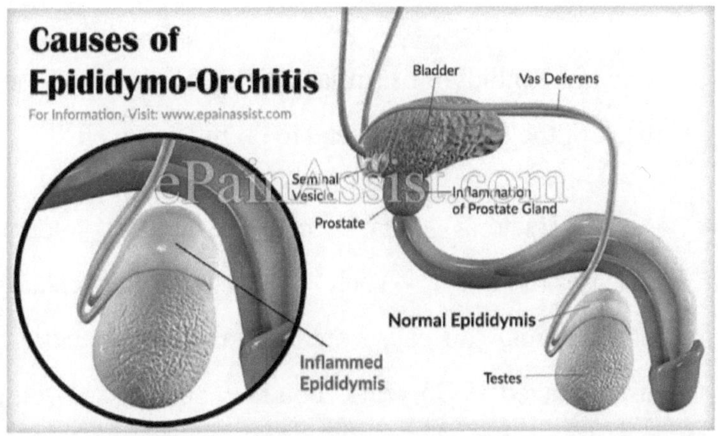

Orchitis is inflammation of one or both testicles in men, usually caused by an infection.

Orchitis can result from the spread of bacteria through the blood from other locations in your body. It also can be a progression of epididymitis, an infection of the tube that carries semen out of the testicles. This is called epididymo-orchitis.

G-2. Orchitis Causes

*   Both bacteria and viruses can cause orchitis.

*   Bacteria that commonly cause orchitis include Escherichia coli, Staphylococcus, and Streptococcus.   A prostate infection may occur in conjunction with orchitis. Epididymitis (inflammation of the tube on the back of the testicle) can lead to orchitis, as well.

*   Bacteria that cause sexually transmitted diseases (STD), such as gonorrhea, chlamydia, and syphilis, can cause orchitis in sexually active men, usually aged 19-35 years. You may be at risk if you have many sexual partners, are involved in high-risk sexual behaviors such as unprotected sex, if your sexual partner has had an STD, or if you have a history of STDs.

*   The virus that causes mumps can cause orchitis, as well. Most common in young boys (rare in boys younger than 10 years), orchitis begins four to six days

after mumps begins. A third of boys with mumps will develop orchitis and end up with a condition called testicular atrophy (shrinking of the testicles). That's why it is so critical for all children, boys especially, to have **shots to protect them from getting the childhood disease of mumps.**

*   You may be at risk for non-sexually transmitted orchitis if you haven't had proper vaccination against mumps, if you get urinary tract infections, if you are older than age 45, or if you frequently have a catheter placed into your bladder.

G-3. Orchitis Symptoms

With orchitis, you may have a rapid onset of pain in one or both testicles that may spread to the groin.

One or both of your testicles may appear tender, swollen, and red or purple.

You might have a "heavy feeling" in the swollen testicle.

You might see blood in your semen.

Other symptoms include high fever, nausea, vomiting, pain with urination, or pain from straining with a bowel movement, groin pain, pain with intercourse, and simply feeling ill.

In epididymo-orchitis, the symptoms are similar and may begin rapidly or progress more gradually.

Orchitis causes a localized area of pain and swelling in the testicle for one to several days.

Later, infection increases to involve the whole testicle.

Possible pain or burning before or after urination and penile discharge are also seen.

G-4. When to Seek Medical Care

Most cases of orchitis caused by bacteria require antibiotics right away. If you suspect that you have the disease, or notice redness, swelling, pain, or inflammation of the scrotum or testicle, call your health care provider immediately. Do not delay medical care.

G-5. Exams and Tests

Your health care provider may perform a series of diagnostic tests.

An ultrasound of the inflamed testicle (or both testicles) can determine the difference between orchitis and testicular torsion, another painful and potentially dangerous condition.

With a rectal exam, your doctor checks your prostate for infection. This test is necessary because antibiotic treatment will be used for a longer period of time if the infection involves the prostate.

A urine sample might be taken to check for STDs and other bacteria that might be responsible for the infection.

Blood is drawn to test for HIV and syphilis if a sexually transmitted disease is suspected.

G-6. Outlook for Orchitis

For some of the men who have orchitis, the affected testicle will shrink and lose its function. The longer you delay getting treatment, the more likely the testicle will have long-term damage. Untreated orchitis can result in infertility, loss of one or both testicles, and severe illness or death.

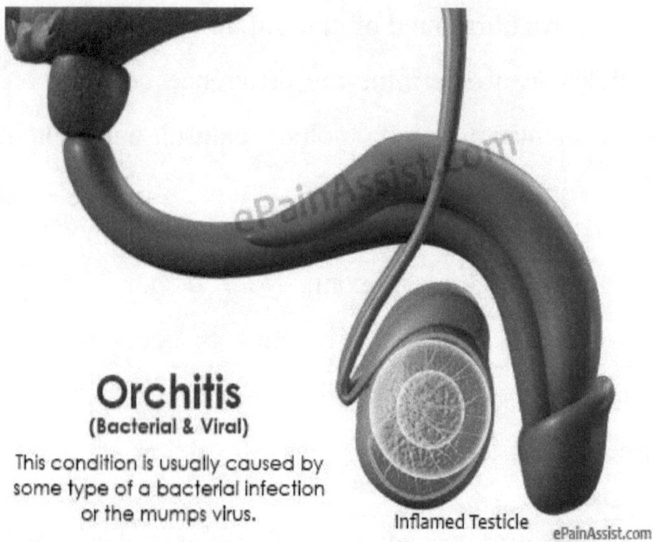

G-7. Most effective Homeopathic medicine for varicoceles Hydrocele Orchitis

Sr. No	Healing Substance	Power	Drops	No. of doses in a day
1	Belladonna	30		
2	Rhododendron	30	2	3
3	Medorrhinum	1 M	2	3
4	Thuja	1 M	2	Morning
5	Echinacea Ang	Q	Mix each of 10 ml in 30 ml of Bottle	20 Drops with ½ Cup of water 3 times a day
6	Calendula	Q		
7	Belladona	Q		

H. Epididymitis

H-1. What Is Epididymitis?

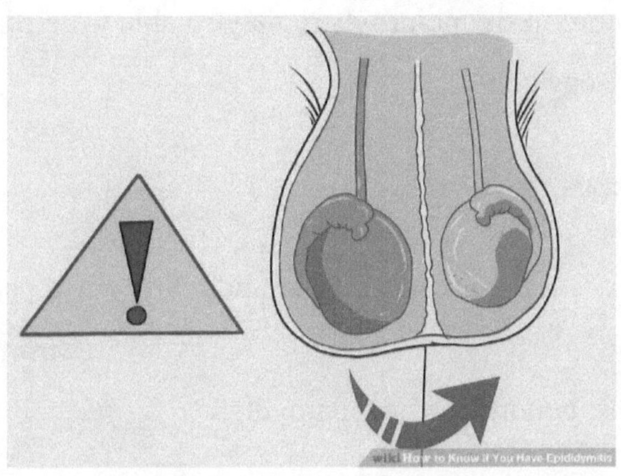

The epididymis -- a long, coiled tube at the back of each of a man's two testicles -- can get inflamed. When that happens, it's called epididymitis.

It's usually caused by a sexually transmitted infection, but several other types of bacteria can cause epididymitis as well.

H-2. What Does the Epididymis Do?

The epididymis carries sperm from the testes, which produce it, to the vas deferens, a tube behind the bladder.

The epididymis lays in coils around the back of a man's testicle and can be nearly 20 feet long.

It can take nearly 2 weeks for sperm to make it from one end of the epididymis to the other. In that time, the sperm cells mature to the point where they're able to fertilize a woman's egg cell.

H-3. Causes

The most common causes of epididymitis are a pair of sexually transmitted infections: gonorrhea and chlamydia.

About 600,000 cases of epididymitis are reported in the United States every year, mostly in men between 18 and 35. In men older than 35, epididymitis usually happens because of an infection of the bladder or urinary tract.

Some cases of epididymitis are caused by the E. coli bacteria, or in rare cases, by the same bacteria that causes tuberculosis.

H-4. Symptoms

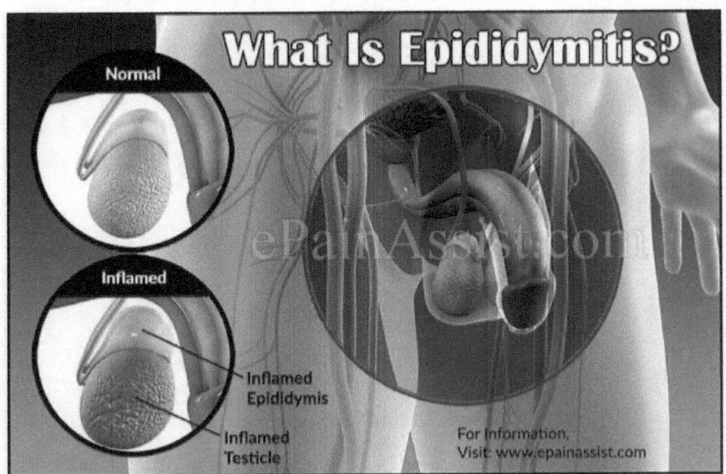

When a bacterial infection strikes, the epididymis gradually becomes swollen and painful. This usually happens on one testicle, rather than both. It can last up to 6 weeks if untreated.

You might have one or more of these other possible symptoms:

- Redness, swelling, or tenderness in the scrotum, the sac that contains the testes
- A more frequent or urgent need to pee
- A lump on your testicle
- Painful urination or ejaculation

- Fever
- Bloody urine
- Discomfort in your lower abdomen
- Enlarged lymph nodes in your groin
- A lump on your testicle
- See your doctor if you have any of these symptoms.

H-5. Related Conditions

Epididymitis shares many of the symptoms of a more serious problem called testicular torsion (that's when a testicle gets turned around the cord that connects it to the body).

Testicular torsion symptoms usually develop much faster, however. Torsion is an emergency that may cause you to lose a testicle if you don't get treatment quickly.

When the swelling and tenderness extends past the epididymis and into the testicle itself, that's known as epididymo-orchitis.

H-6. Diagnosis and Tests

When you go to the doctor, he will examine your scrotum for signs of infection and ask you questions about your symptoms. He might also do a rectal exam to check your prostate and check for any tenderness.

1. If your doctor suspects epididymitis based on the exam, you might get one or more tests. They include:
2. Urine sample: You may pee into a cup so a lab can check for signs of an infection.
3. Blood sample: This can also find abnormalities.
4. Swab sample: For this test, your doctor inserts a narrow swab into the tip of your penis to get a sample of discharge. This is used to test for chlamydia or gonorrhea.
5. Ultrasound: You might also be asked to sit for an ultrasound test, which uses sound waves to produce an image of your scrotum and testicles.

H-7. Possible Complications

If left untreated, epididymitis can become a "chronic" condition, one that lingers and causes recurring problems.

Epididymitis might also cause in infection in the scrotum.

H-8. Tell Your Partners

If your condition is the result of a sexually transmitted disease, you should tell anyone with whom you have had sex in the past 60 days about your diagnosis. If it's been more than 60 days since you had sex, contact your most recent sex partner.

They should see a doctor and get tested for sexually transmitted diseases as well.

Top of Form

H-9. Most effective Homeopathic medicine for Epididymitis

Sr. No	Healing Substance	Power	No. of Drops	Daily Dose
1	Thuja	1 M	2	Night
2	Rhododendron	30	2	Afternoon
3	chrysanthemum	1 M	2	3
4	Apis mellifica	30	2	Morning
5	Calcarea fluorica	6 x	6 Tab	3 Times

Use these effective remedies about Seven to Thirteen Months for Complete Healing & check up after every 3 Months.

Infertility involving Spermatorrhoea

The meaning of Spermatorrhea is the flow of semen with urine. In such cases, semen passes either while passing urine or while passing stool when straining due to constipation. In few cases, the semen passes even before urination or also mixed with urine. In Spermatorrhea, the semen is secreted from testicles. It has also been noticed that some time instead of semen, secretion is passed from the prostate, which is known as prostatorrhea. The secretion from the prostate is milky without Spermatozoa while on the other hand in semen, spermatozoa are present.

This can be checked by the help of microscope. Over and above, sometimes the secretions take place from vesicles or Cowper's glands. The secretion of vesicles is yellow in color and that of Cowper's glands is colorless like water.

However, if prostatorrhea is not checked may cause Spermatorrhea. Therefore, this ailment should not be ignored at all and should be treated as soon as possible since it disturbs the whole nervous system and may cause impotency.

Symptoms of Spermatorrhea

Observed symptoms are many and visible; it includes weakness of sight, dizziness, high heart bit rate and dyspepsia. Also back pain, fatigue, incapability of mental effort and sometimes chest tremors are detected. While this list is this long, often most of it relapses on their own meaning it is all mild and temporary. It becomes psychological though and depression is the perfect choice because the victim is simply shunning away from everybody like as if everybody knows his problem.

The condition is really a symptom and not a disease; it does not in itself precipitate in to a disease demanding treatment. It emanates from the gonads though but it ends up being a weak nervous system requiring attention.

Homeopathic medicines for Spermatorrhea

Homeopathy is one of the most popular holistic systems of medicine. The selection of remedy is based upon the theory of individualization and symptoms similarity by using holistic approach. This is the only way through which a state of complete health can be regained by removing all the sign and symptoms from which the patient is suffering. The aim of homeopathy is not only to treat Spermatorrhea but to address its underlying cause and individual susceptibility. As far as therapeutic medication is concerned, several remedies are available to treat Spermatorrhea that can be selected on the basis of cause, sensations and modalities of the complaints. For individualized remedy selection and treatment, the patient should consult a qualified homeopathic doctor in person. There are following remedies which are helpful in the treatment of Spermatorrhea:

Agnus castus – loss of both sexual desire and erection with coldness of the sexual organs; sometimes scanty emission without ejaculation and sometimes great loss of semen during sleep with lack of courage; nervous depression and mental weakness. Sexual melancholy with pains; organ cold and relaxed with physical weakness.

Picric acid – Spermatorrhea with great sexual desire followed by prostration; involuntary seminal emission during sleep without sensual dreams followed by great weakness.

Phosphoric acid – remarkable remedy for Spermatorrhea associated with general irritability, distressed and anxious with burning in the spine, penis has no power of erection, along with all this, the scrotum and testicles are flabby.

Selenium – more suitable for seminal emissions, voluntary or involuntary, associated with an increased desire and decreased ability; sexual thoughts accompanied by dribbling of semen during sleep and loss of sexual power; on attempting coition, the penis becomes relaxed with the feeling of sexual neurasthenia.

Staphysagria – is the remedy for the bad effects of masturbation where there is great emaciation with dark rings under the eyes, sallow face, peevishness and shyness. The patient is hypochondriacal and permits the mind to dwell too long on sexual subjects; the boy becomes apathetic and gloomy, he has the sunken face and he becomes uneasy about the state of his health.

There may also be irritability of the prostatic portion of the urethra.

Conium – this remedy, on account of its mental conditions, is of a great utility in the treatment of sexual excess. Spermatorrhea from long lasting abuse of genital organs, face pale and sunken, with blue rings around the eyes; dread of company, yet does not want to be alone.

Sulphur – there is frequent involuntary emission of semen at night without any erection of the penis. The seminal flow is thin and watery.

Useful when the patient feels weakness, suffers from gastric ailments and the genital organs relaxed, the penis is cold, the erections are few; lasting a short while. In coitus, the semen escapes too soon, almost at the first contact.

Cantharis – seminal emission at night, followed by a disagreeable burning heat all over body, great anxiety, heaviness, inability to sleep for the rest of the night; nightly emissions followed by shivering lasting for an hour or two and sleeplessness for that night; partial blindness for an self to work and thus life becomes a burden; violent painful priapism, discharge of blood instead of semen.

Cina Officinalis – more suitable for the acute effects, such as emissions on three or four consecutive nights weakening the patient greatly. Spermatorrhea with excited, lascivious and fancy dreams at night associated with debility from exhausting discharge.

Calcaria Carb – bad effects of early masturbation; night sweats follow every emission, or, after marriage, every coitus is followed by weakness of mind and body; increased sexual desire provokes emission, but unusual weakness follows indulgence, and ejaculations is tardy; burning and stinging while semen discharges during coition; pressing pain in head and back; lassitude and weakness in lower extremities; sweats easily.

Nux Vomica – for the bad effects of early masturbation; it should ne give when the patient suffers from headache, frequent involuntary emissions at night, especially toward morning, and the digestive organs are weak. There is an irritable condition from sexual excess, erections taking place, but they are not under the control of the mind and may subside at any time during an embrace; this is a common complaint of city man who have been high lives and drinkers all their lives.

Caladium – here, after masturbation, the penis is as flabby as a rag, the prepuce when withdrawn behind the glans does not have sufficient contractility to replace itself. Nocturnal emission occurs with or without dreams. It is indicated in the advanced stages when there are no erections. Emissions occurring without any sexual excitement whatever is a good indication for caladium. Feeling of coldness and cold perspiration about the genitals is also a useful symptom for the remedy.

Zincum –This remedy corresponds to long-lasting abuse of the genital organs, with great hypochondriasis. The patient has a pale sunken face with blue rings about the eyes, and there is with this drug great local local irritation, the testicles being drawn up against the external ring. Aurum may be useful when despondency predominates.

Lycopodium – Lycopodium is the remedy for cases which have gone on to complete impotency; the erections are absent or imperfect and the genital organs are cold and shrivelled. Exhausting pollutions (Nocturnal

Emissions or Wet Dreams) in men without erections. Lilienthal termed Lycopodium "the old man's balm." It corresponds especially to the impotency of old age where there is great despondency. Kobalt has backache following seminal emissions. Sarsaparilla has nocturnal erections with lascivious dreams, followed by pain in the back down to the spermatic cords; prostration, the least excitement causing ejaculation without sexual feeling.

Most effective Homeopathic medicine for **Spermatorrhoea**

Sr. No	Healing Substance	Power	No. of Drops	Daily Dose
1	Selenium	6x,12x or 30	3	3
2	Agnus Castus	6x,12x or 30	3	3
3	Nuphar luteum	30	2	3
4	Nux Vomika	30	2	3
5	Staphisagria	30	2	3

Thanking You.